Supporting Families with a Child with a Disability

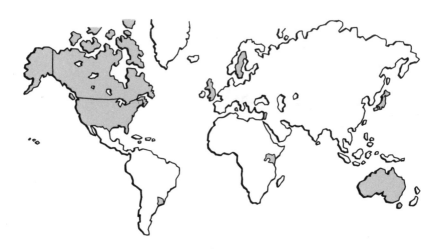

Supporting Families with a Child with a Disability

An International Outlook

by

Alan Gartner, Ph.D.
Professor and Director
Office of Sponsored Research
The Graduate School and University Center
The City University of New York
New York, New York

Dorothy Kerzner Lipsky, Ph.D.
Assistant Superintendent
Oceanside (NY) Public Schools and
Senior Research Scientist
Office of Sponsored Research
The Graduate School and University Center
The City University of New York
New York, New York

and

Ann P. Turnbull, Ed.D.
Co-Director
Beach Center on Families and Disability and
Professor
University of Kansas
Lawrence, Kansas

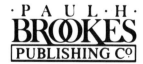

·P A U L·H·
BROOKES
PUBLISHING CO.

Baltimore • London • Toronto • Sydney

Paul H. Brookes Publishing Co.
P.O. Box 10624
Baltimore, Maryland 21285-0624

Copyright © 1991 by Paul H. Brookes Publishing Co., Inc.
All rights reserved.

Typeset by The Composing Room of Michigan, Inc., Grand Rapids,
Michigan.
Manufactured in the United States of America by
The Maple Press Company, York, Pennsylvania.

Library of Congress Cataloging-in-Publication Data
Gartner, Alan.
  Supporting families with a child with a disability : an
international outlook / Alan Gartner, Dorthy Kerzner
Lipsky, Ann P. Turnbull.
      p. cm.
  Includes bibliographical references and index.
  ISBN 1-55766-059-X
  1. Family social work—Cross-cultural studies—
Congresses. 2. Parents of handicapped children—
Services for—Cross-cultural studies—Congresses. 3.
Aid to families with dependent children programs—
Cross-cultural studies—Congresses. I. Lipsky, Dorothy
Kerzner. II. Turnbull, Ann P., 1947–   . III. Title.
HV697.G37 1990
362.82′8–dc20   90-2266
                                                       CIP

Contents

Preface vii
Acknowledgments xiii
National Teams xv
Conference Participants xvii

Chapter 1 Introduction 1
Chapter 2 Culture and Disability 17
Chapter 3 Families and a Child with a Disability 57
Chapter 4 Basic Social Welfare Provisions
          and Financial Assistance 97
Chapter 5 Informing Families 127
Chapter 6 Education 137
Chapter 7 Taking a Break from Responsibility
          for Meeting the Child's Needs 155
Chapter 8 Emotional Support 165
Chapter 9 Employment, Housing, and Recreation 175
Chapter 10 Conclusion 185
Afterword 213
Index 225

Preface

This book is concerned with three entwined issues—disability, culture, and family—and the ways in which they play themselves out in the lives of families with a child with a disability. While based upon specific activities in nine countries across the globe, it is in keeping with a book whose production crossed the turn of the decade from the 1980s to the 1990s that the issues are changing, indeed, emerging. As we discuss in Chapter 2, the understanding of the meaning of disability varies in the context of differing cultures and is continually shifting; at the same time, there is an emerging sense of a culture of disability that crosses national boundaries.[1]

There is changing understanding of family, including its make-up and functions, as we discuss in Chapter 3. Throughout the world, as shifts occur in basic economic conditions—the move in some areas from an agricultural to an industrialized society, and in others from an industrialized to a post-industrial or service society—there are changes in the family, in the roles of both the family as a unit and its individual members.

"In the past, a family was seen as an economic unit, important for economic exchanges, such as inheritances. In contemporary times, families have been perceived as a psychological unit" (Voydanoff, cited in Gustis, 1989, p. C6). And, more broadly, Turnbull and colleagues (1985) have emphasized a family sys-

---

[1]Important here is the development of links across countries of persons with disabilities. Note, for example, the establishment of Disabled Peoples' International (Miller & Chadderdon, 1982). In addition, of course, there are inter-national organizations concerned with persons with disabilities, such as the International League of Societies for Persons with Mental Handicap, as well as organizations concerned with international exchanges, such as Rehabilitation International, UNICEF, the World Institute on Disability, and the World Rehabilitation Fund. Pertinent, too, is the United Nations decade of disabled persons (1983–1992) activities (*World Programmes*, 1983). A special issue of *Disability Studies Quarterly*, edited by Groce (1987), offers a rare cross-cultural perspective.

tems approach. In the United States, for example, in 1970, 40% of families fit the traditional definition of two parents living with children; by 1988 this was true of only 27% of families. Here, as in Chapter 2, we rely primarily upon data and examples from the United States. We do so, not in the belief that it is representative of the world as a whole, but rather because in the field of disability its practices are often considered a standard for the rest of the world. As indicated throughout the book, we believe that this is not the only standard and is not necessarily the best standard. Moreover, in the heart of the book, Chapters 4 through 9, data and examples are drawn from all nine countries.

While the industrialized and wealthy countries provide a wider range of formal services, this does not always result in better support for families. Indeed, in many countries, Canada for example, there is an effort to move away from formal service provision to greater use of informal systems and natural environments. However, in less wealthy countries, Kenya for example, there are increasing efforts to develop government provided services. Another area of contrasting development is the extent to which services for people with disabilities are organized separately from the general social service system. Sweden is at least a partial resolution to this dichotomy of services, with the primary design there involving the incorporation of services to persons with disabilities as part of the "regular" services to various population groups, for example, children, families, workers, and so forth.

While there is great diversity among the nine countries, there are some apparent common developments or trends. These include:

- A growing sense that persons with disabilities[2] can and should live in the community and not in institutional settings
- The growth of national legislation to provide increased services to persons with disabilities, especially children

---

[2]We embrace the distinctions made by the World Health Organization among impairment, disability, and handicap. *Impairment:* Any loss or abnormality of psychological, physiological, or anatomical structure or function. *Disability:* any restriction or lack (resulting from an impairment) of ability to

- The development of rights-based guarantees, both to persons with disabilities and (to a lesser extent) to their families, of participation in decisions affecting them
- The belief that the environment, physical and social, is the key factor that determines the extent to which an individual's impairment becomes a handicap
- A recognition that the family, in both the attitudes it has and the support it receives, is the central social institution affecting the life of the child with disabilities
- Increasing development of organizations among persons with disabilities, parents of children with disabilities, and other interested groups, including professionals; there is, however, generally little in the way of collaboration among these groups.

The nine countries represented at the Wingspread Conference span the globe, as the map at the beginning of the book indicates. They are not, of course, representative of the world at large; they are more of an opportunity sample. However, as the data in Tables 1 and 2 indicate, they do vary a good deal in terms of size, population, density, wealth, age of the population, and infant mortality. Notably absent from the table are data about persons with disabilities. Given the differing definitions and various collection schemes, there are no good comparative data, indeed little good data in any individual country.[3]

While in each of the countries there is recognition that among its different cultural groups there are varying understandings of and responses to disability, nonetheless, there

---

perform an activity in the manner or within the range considered normal for a human being. *Handicap:* A disadvantage for a given individual, resulting from an impairment or disability, that limits or prevents the fulfillment of a role that is normal, depending on age, sex, social, and cultural factors, for that individual (World Health Organization, 1980).

[3]The United Nations estimates that there are 500 million persons with disabilities worldwide. "In most countries, at least one person in 10 is disabled by physical, mental, or sensory impairment, and at least 25% of the population is adversely affected by the presence of disability" (*World Programmes*, 1983, p. 11). The figures in nonindustrial countries are as high as 20% and 50%, respectively (p. 13). Acton (1987) points out that two-thirds of those with disabilities "needed assistance they could not get for the simple reason that the required services did not exist where they live" (p. 35).

Table 1. National comparisons by size and population

Country	Square miles	Physical size Population/ square mile	% Urban	Population
Australia	2,966,200	5	85%	16,090,000
Canada	3,851,790	6	75%	25,334,000
Israel	7,847	570	89%	4,477,000
Japan	145,856	844	76%	123,231,000
Kenya	224,960	105	16%	23,727,000
Sweden	173,731	48	85%	8,371,000
U.K.	94,226	601	92%	56,648,000
U.S.A.	3,618,770	68	79%	247,498,000
Uruguay	68,037	43	86%	2,983,000

Table 2. National comparisons by wealth, age, and infant mortality

Country	Wealth GNP	Per capita	Age 0–14	15–59	60+	Infant mortality (per 1000)
Australia	$ 153 B	$10,282	23%	62%	15%	9
Canada	367 B	13,000	22%	63%	15%	8
Israel	25 B	5,995	33%	55%	12%	13
Japan	1,900 B	10,266	20%	64%	16%	6
Kenya	6 B	322	52%	43%	5%	83
Sweden	100 B	11,989	18%	59%	23%	3
U.K.	453 B	7,216	19%	60%	21%	10
U.S.A.	4,200 B	13,451	22%	62%	16%	10
Uruguay	5 B	1,665	27%	58%	15%	26

B = Billion

appears to be little in the way of systematic national efforts to attune policies and services to these differences.[4] The ethnocentrism here is but a reflection of the larger picture in which the needs of minorities are subject to the dominance of the value system of the majority. Social service systems are both the instrument and the reflection of national values in general. This is true, specifically, in terms of the services provided to support families with a child with a disability.

---

[4]A notable development in this area is the existence of a special office for minority affairs in Australia.

REFERENCES

Acton, N. (1987). Classics revisited. *Disability Studies Quarterly, 7* (3), 34–37.

Groce, N. (1987). Cross-cultural research: Current strengths, future needs. *Disability Studies Quarterly, 7*(3), 1–3.

Gustis, P.S. (1989, August 31). What is a family? Traditional limits are being withdrawn. *New York Times,* p. C1, 6.

Miller, K.S., & Chadderdon, L.M. (1982). *A voice of our own: Proceedings of the First World Congress of Disabled Peoples' International.* East Lansing, MI: University Center for International Rehabilitation, Michigan State University.

Turnbull, A.P., Brotherson, M.J., & Summers, A.J. (1985). The impact of deinstitutionalization on families: A family systems approach. In R.H. Bruininks & K.C. Lakin (Eds.), *Living and learning in the least restrictive environment* (pp. 115–140). Baltimore: Paul H. Brookes Publishing Co.

World Health Organization. (1980). *International classifications of impairments, disabilities, and handicaps.* Geneva, Switzerland: Author.

World programmes of action concerning disabled persons: United Nations decade of disabled persons, 1983–1992. New York: The United Nations.

Acknowledgments

This book is the second product of "A Cross-Cultural Conference on Supports for Families with a Child with a Disability," held at the Johnson Foundation's Wingspread Conference Center in Racine, Wisconsin, June, 1988. National teams from Australia, Canada, Israel, Japan, Kenya, Sweden, the United Kingdom, the United States, and Uruguay participated in the conference. The first product, *Supports for Families with a Disabled Child: Collected Papers from an International Cross-Cultural Conference* (1989), presented the papers prepared for the conference by eight (the team from Sweden was not included) of the national teams. That volume describes the situations in those countries and is the product of its papers' authors.

In this volume the focus and the responsibility are different. Our goals are both to examine the concept of family support in a cross-cultural and cross-national context and to present its characteristics, comparing and contrasting developments in the nine countries. Toward these goals, we draw upon the papers presented at the Wingspread conference,[1] the discussion there, and additional material. While responsibility is ours, the listing of the authors of these papers on page xv is acknowledgment of their contribution; here, we want to express our appreciation to them for their work and collaboration. Also, we are grateful to the other participants[2] at the Wingspread conference who helped to make it such a productive and enjoyable event.

Additionally, we are grateful to the sponsors of the conference: The Graduate School and University Center of The City University of New York, The World Institute on Disability (especially Judy Heumann), The World Rehabilitation Fund (especially Diane Woods), and we thank the people at Wingspread (especially Dick Kinch and the late Kay Mauer). Finally, we are grateful to the International League of Societies for Persons with Mental Handicap (especially its President, Eloisa de Lorenzo, and its Family Committee, chaired by Ann P. Turnbull), which co-sponsored the conference and supported the production of this book. We are pleased to contribute the royalties from the book to support the work of the League's 113 Societies in 76 countries.

---

[1]For the reader's convenience, we will not generally use quotation marks or footnotes for this material. Unless otherwise indicated, the material in Chapters 4–9 about the situation in each country is drawn from *Supports for Families with a Disabled Child* (1989).

[2]In addition to the teams from the nine countries, delegations from Tanzania and Uganda were present. Among the 39 participants, nine were parents of children with disabilities and four were themselves persons with disabilities.

xiii

National Teams

Australia

Judy Ellis
Doug Limbrick
Silvana Scibilia
Jenny Sharples

Canada

Bruce Kappel
Evelyn Lusthaus
Judith Snow

Israel

Victor Florian
Shlomo Katz

Japan

Fusako Oi
Keiko Higuchi
Ko Takei

Kenya

Aloys A. Odeck

Sweden

Gunilla Roden
Inger Claesson Wastberg
Ann-Marie Wendelholt

United Kingdom

Peter Mittler
Philippa Russell

United States

John Agosta
Judy Cohen
Shirley Cohen
Rachel Warren

Uruguay

Rodolfo Speranza

Conference Participants

John M. Agosta
Research Associate
Human Services Research
  Institute
2336 Massachusetts Avenue
Cambridge, Massachusetts
  02140
U.S.A.

Melissa A. Behm
Vice President
Paul H. Brookes Publishing
  Company
Post Office Box 10624
Baltimore, Maryland 21285
U.S.A.

David Braddock
Professor of Community Health
  Sciences
Institute for the Study of
  Developmental Disabilities
University of Illinois at Chicago
1640 West Roosevelt Road
Chicago, Illinois 60608
U.S.A.

Judith Cohen
Director of Utilization/Education
The Institutes of Applied Human
  Dynamics
3625 Bainbridge Avenue
Bronx, New York 10467
U.S.A.

Shirley Cohen
Associate Dean
Division of Programs in
  Education
Hunter College
The City University of New York
Room 1000 West
695 Park Avenue
New York, New York 10021
U.S.A.

Lorraine Cole
Director
Office of Minority Concerns
American Speech-Language-
  Hearing Association
10801 Rockville Pike
Rockville, Maryland 20852
U.S.A.

Harold Cox
Doctoral Student
Florence Heller School
Brandeis University
208 Ridge Street
Winchester, Massachusetts
  01890
U.S.A.

Victor Florian
Senior Lecturer
Department of Psychology
Bar Ilan University
52100 Ramat-Gan
Israel

Alan Gartner
Professor and Director
Office of Sponsored Research
The Graduate School and
  University Center
The City University of New York
33 West 42nd Street
New York, New York 10036
U.S.A.

Nora Groce
Research Associate
Boston Children's Hospital
Harvard University
300 Longwood Avenue
Box 23
Boston, Massachusetts 02115
U.S.A.

Judith E. Heumann
Co-Director
World Institute on Disability
1720 Oregon Street
Berkeley, California 94703
U.S.A.

Keiko Higuchi
Coordinator
The Human Care Association
178-3 Negishi-cho
Machida-City
Tokyo 194
Japan

Francine H. Jacobs
Assistant Professor
Eliot-Pearson Department of
   Child Study
Tufts University
Medford, Massachusetts 02155
U.S.A.

Jill Kagan
Professional Staff
Select Committee on Children,
   Youth and Families
United States House of
   Representatives
Room 385, HOB Annex 2
2nd & D Streets, SW
Washington, DC 20515
U.S.A.

Bruce Kappel
Principal
Kappel Consulting
91 Southill Drive
Don Mills, Ontario M3C 2H9
Canada

Naomi Karp
Program Specialist
National Institute on Disability
   and Rehabilitation Research
United States Department of
   Education
400 Maryland Avenue, SW
Mail Stop 2305
Washington, DC 20202
U.S.A.

Shlomo Katz
Associate Professor
Department of Psychology
Coordinator
Rehabilitation Psychology
   Program
Bar Ilan University
52100 Ramat-Gan
Israel

Doug Limbrick
Director
Supported Accommodation
   Program
Australian Department of
   Community Services and
   Health
G.P.O. Box 9848
Canberra ACT 2601
Australia

Jane S. Lin-Fu
Acting Chief
Maternal and Child Health
   Resource Development
United States Public Health
   Service
5600 Fishers Lane
Rockville, Maryland 20857
U.S.A.

Dorothy Kerzner Lipsky
Co-Chairperson
Senior Research Scientist
The Graduate School and
   University Center
The City University of New York
Room 1610
33 West 42nd Street
New York, New York 10036
U.S.A.

Elizabeth Madraa
Senior Medical Officer
Ministry of Health, Uganda
Hubert H. Humphrey Fellowship
   Program
New York State College of
   Agriculture and Life Sciences

Cornell University
Roberts Hall
Post Office Box 16
Ithaca, New York 14853–5901
U.S.A.

Peter J. Mittler
Professor of Special Education
Centre for Educational Guidance
  and Special Needs
University of Manchester
Oxford Road
Manchester M13 9PL
England

Alois Odeck
Member, Board of Directors
Civitan Foundation
Post Office Box 42371
Nairobi
Kenya

Fusako Oi
Chief of Research Section
The Kanagawa Medical and
  Welfare Foundation for
  Children
1-9-1 Nishikanagawa
Kanagawa-Ku
Yokohama 221
Japan

Gunilla Roden
Nordostra Omsorgsomradet
  (ONO)
Soltorpsvagen 16
Box 520
18215 Danderyd
Sweden

Anne Rosewater
Staff Director
Select Committee on Children,
  Youth and Families
United States House of
  Representatives
Room 385 HOB, Annex 2
2nd & D Streets, SW
Washington, DC 20515
U.S.A.

Philippa Russell
Research Officer
Voluntary Council for
  Handicapped Children
8 Wakley Street
London ECIV 7QE
England

Silvana C. Scibilia
Director
Action on Disability Within
  Ethnic Communities
123–125 Sydney Road
Brunswick
Victoria 3056
Australia

Rodolfo Speranza
Health and Sanitary Advisor in
  the Field of Rehabilitation
Ministry of Public Health
c/o Eloisa de Lorenza
Buschental 3347
Montevideo
Uruguay

Susan Sygall
Executive Director
Mobility International USA
Post Office Box 3551
Eugene, Oregon 97403
U.S.A.

Kou Takei
Vocation Social Worker
Section of Community
  Resources Development
Kanagawa-Ken Social Welfare
  Council
Sawatari 4-2
Kanagawa-Ku
Yokohama-Shi
Kanagawa-Ken
Japan

Setsuko Tsuj
Interpreter
The Human Care Association
1614 24th Street
Sacramento, California 95816
U.S.A.

Frida D. Tungaraza
Special Education Department
The Ohio State University
356 Arps Hall
1945 North High Street
Columbus, Ohio 43210–1172
U.S.A.

Ann P. Turnbull
Co-Chairperson
Professor
Beach Center on Families and
    Disability
University of Kansas
2045 Haworth Hall
Lawrence, Kansas 66045
U.S.A.

Rachel D. Warren
Director
National Resource Center on
    Family Based Services
School of Social Work
University of Iowa
N240 Oakdale Hall
Oakdale, Iowa 52319
U.S.A.

Inger Claesson Wastberg
Director
Institute for Integration
Norrmalmstorg 1,
S-111 46 Stockholm
Sweden

Ann-Marie Wendelholt
Ombudsman
The Swedish Society for the
    Mentally Handicapped
Lansforbundet FUB
Vardcentrum
S-534 00 Vara
Sweden

Maureen West
Professional Staff Member
Office of Senator Lowell Weicker
United States Senate
Russell Building 225
Washington, DC 20510
U.S.A.

Diane E. Woods
Project Director
World Rehabilitation Fund
International Exchange of
    Experts and Information in
    Rehabilitation
400 East 34th Street
New York, New York 10016
U.S.A.

Supporting Families with a Child with a Disability

1

Introduction

Where imagery leads, policy follows, and behavior results. (Goodman, 1989, p. 58)

What does it mean to have a disability? Through what—and whose—lens is disability seen? Indeed, who is disabled?[1] What does it mean to provide support for a family? What is a family—nuclear or extended, whole or "broken" (whatever that might mean)? Indeed, should support provided go to the abstraction called a "family" or to the individual persons it includes, for the different needs of each?

Across these sets of questions, another fundamental question exists: What is special about a family with a member with a disability? Are the needs of persons (including children) called disabled different from the needs of others? And whatever these differences, should society's response be different for subgroups of the general population?

These are fundamental issues. A full discussion of them is beyond the scope of this book, but these issues are central to its

---

[1] In this text and elsewhere, we treat persons with disabilities as a single group. In fact, we recognize that they are both individuals and also members of many subcategories. At the same time, they are in many ways a single group, especially in the way public policies treat them.

1

concerns. Our focus is on families with a child with a disability. In this and the following chapter, we examine the ways in which society considers and treats persons designated as disabled; indeed, we consider the bases and ways of designation. The circle of imagery, policy, and behavior that Goodman expressed in the quotation that begins this chapter is nicely captured by Giami (1987), writing about the treatment of persons with mental retardation in France. "A large proportion of specialised institutions for the mentally retarded are closed ones with limited relationships with the outside world. The extreme protection afforded to the disabled can in some cases constitute an ideological rationalisation of their exclusion" (p. 45).

While in Chapters 3 through 9 we address the issues as they concern children with disabilities, the focus in this and the following chapter is upon adults with disabilities. This is for two reasons. First, the majority of research about persons with disabilities is focused on adults; second, the current treatment of children with disabilities by professionals, as well as the attitudinal milieu in which they live, is a reflection of the treatment of adults with disabilities.

In contemporary society, there is increasing emphasis on a culturally loaded sense of bodily perfection. This places people—especially children—in the position of having to meet someone else's standards of "perfection," which ultimately is an untenable position. Furthermore, this emphasis does not prepare parents (or children) to deal with the vicissitudes of life. Finally, the emphasis on bodily perfection—or the absence of imperfection or impairment—leads to ignoring the growing recognition that impairments become handicaps as a result of societal response, both environmental and social.

The lives of persons with impairments, especially children,[2] are not set in fixed and immutable arcs but are open to a range of opportunity, limited less by the impairments than by societal attitudes that result in the absence of supports for these persons and their families. The determination of these attitudes is a consequence of the way people view others, including those with disabilities. Goffman (1963) captures this

---

[2]Coles (1979) captures this in a quote by a young woman with polio about her plans for the future: "I want to live my life! And I will!" (p. ix). He expresses something of the problems that people with disabilities face, in the language of those who sympathize with them, noting that his inquiries, ironically, were "arrogant, condescending, and blind [sic] . . . " (p. ix).

point, stating, "Society establishes the means of categorizing persons and the complement of attributes felt to be ordinary and natural for members of each of these categories" (p. 2). Edgerton (1970) makes the point just as succinctly: "Any social system can make any behavior into a social problem" (p. 525).

In part, the way people categorize others is a function of the lens through which people look at individual attributes. And such lenses vary—over time, place and culture, and discipline. In Chapter 2, we examine some of these differences in terms of time and culture. A publication of the Australian government reflects a different lens, presenting alternatives to traditional myths about disability (see the Appendix to this chapter). Some differences in terms of discipline[3] are noted below:

> Psychological analyses tend to regard it [disability] as an individual experience, with an eye to understanding how physical and mental limitations interact with personality development. Economic analyses treat disability as a social position with its own income stream, much like a job, and seek to explain the extent to which individual choice determines the assumption of the disabled role. Sociological analyses focus on the institutions that treat, house, and manage disabled people—including families, schools, hospitals and rehabilitation clinics—and above all, they examine disability as a stigmatized social status, exploring the means by which stigma is created, maintained, and resisted.
>
> [A] political approach . . . explore[s] the meaning of disability for the state—the formal institutions of government, and the intellectual justifications that give coherence to their activities. . . . Why does the state create a category of disability in the first place, and how does it design a workable administrative definition? (Stone, 1984, pp. 3–4)

No one of these lenses is "better" than another, nor do they operate in isolation from one another. For example, the ways in which the state behaves—the subject of a political analysis—are both the causes and consequences of the attitudes (including stigma) that a sociological approach examines (Gartner & Joe, 1987).

Sociologists look not at the person of the deviator but at the process of deviance:

> Social groups create deviance by making the rules whose infraction constitutes deviance, and by applying these rules to particular people and labeling them as outsiders. From this point of view,

---

[3]Of course, it is necessary to note that these disciplines of contemporary "Western" society are bound by its fetters.

> deviance is *not* [italics in the original] a quality of the act the person commits, but rather the consequence of the application by others of rules and sanctions to an "offender". The deviant is one to whom that label has successfully been applied; deviant behavior is behavior that people so label. (Becker, 1963, p. 9)

This is also explained in Bogdan and Taylor's (1982) discussion of mental retardation:

> As a concept, mental retardation exists in the minds of those who use it as a term to describe the cognitive states of other people. It is a reification—a socially created category which is assumed to have an existence independent of its creators' minds. (p. 7)

Haywood (1970) makes a connection to cultural factors: "The variability in individual levels of adjustment-mental competence that is tolerated without assigning deviant status to individuals depends to a large extent upon the demands and customs of the particular culture" (p. 771). In a pathbreaking study, Scott (1969) demonstrates how through the instrument of the agencies it establishes to serve them, society "makes" blind people.

> The disability of blindness is a learned social role. The various attitudes and patterns of behavior that characterize people who are blind are not inherent in their condition but rather are acquired through ordinary processes of social learning. Thus there is nothing inherent in the condition of blindness that requires a person to be dependent, melancholy or helpless; nor is there anything about it that should lead him [sic] to become independent or assertive. Blind men are made, and by the same processes of socialization that have made us all. (p. 14)

Most analyses focus on the negative consequences of such categorization; however, Stone (1984) points out:

> Disability functions as a privileged category [in that] the state accords special treatment to some people who are disabled. Disability accounts for a substantial portion of income distribution and, in much smaller measure, for the distribution of some privileges and [excusing persons so labelled from certain] duties of citizenship—the obligation to serve in national defense, to obey the laws of the state, and to honor financial agreements. (p. 4)

While Stone accurately describes these privileges and the excusing of persons with disabilities from certain duties, she fails to note that there is a cost to such "benefits," namely a perpetuation of the image of incapacity. Perhaps this is so because her lens is political while the cost is largely psychological.

Stone focuses on how societies address the distributive dilemma—the tension between systems based upon work and those based upon need.

> To resolve it, society must develop a set of rules to determine the boundaries of the two systems, rules that specify who is subject to each distributive principle and what is to be distributed within each system. There is no natural boundary between the two systems, no inherent definition of what constitutes need or who "belongs" in one system or the other. Rather, the boundary is something that each society has to invent, to redesign in the face of changing social conditions, and to enforce. Different societies will find different resolutions at different periods of their history. A successful resolution will have certain general characteristics, but every particular resolution is designed by politics, not by some universal logic. (p. 17)

> The concept of disability is fundamentally the result of political conflict about distributive criteria and the appropriate recipients of social aid. Instead of seeing disability as a set of objective characteristics that render people needy, we can define it in terms of ideas and values about distribution. A political analysis must therefore begin by elucidating the dimensions of the disability concept that give it legitimacy as a distributive criterion. (p. 172)

Contemporary welfare states have resolved the distributive dilemma by giving dominance to the primary distributive system—the one based upon work—by granting categorical exemptions from the labor market. This is done using principles such as age (youth or old age) and sickness (or disability).

> Each category must be based on a culturally legitimate rationale for nonparticipation in the labor system. Since the dominant ideology in a market society holds that each individual is responsible for fulfilling his or her needs by working and earning, categories will define conditions under which people cannot be held responsible for working. The traditional categories have been childhood, old age, sickness, and sometimes widowhood. The rationale behind these categories is that something inherent in the conditions they describe *prevents* [italics in the original] people from working, no matter how strong the will to work in individual cases. The categories are meant to describe circumstances under which individuals cannot be held at fault for not working. (Stone, 1984, p. 22)

In a sense, these "objective" categories of age (and sickness or disability) have differing meanings. Thus, for example, the incorporation in the United States Social Security system of retirement at age 65, or more precisely, of the distributive dilemma of eligibility, is not a matter of capacity to work but an historical accident—namely, the copying of the German retirement age. Indeed, the former Commissioner of the Social Security Administration has argued that, "If 65 was the proper retirement age in the U.S. in 1940, then today, based on rising life expectancy, it should be 73" (Hardy, 1989, A8). And Stone (1984) notes that "there is blindness and there is 'legal blindness'. . . . [L]egal blindness is a socially created category, established for specific policy purposes as part of the general categorical resolution of the distributive dilemma" (p. 27).

In contemporary Western society, by the use of the political "lens" the distributive dilemma is resolved based upon automatic entitlement to social aid on the bases of old age, childhood, and disability. However, one needs to go beyond the use of the political lens alone. As the author of a study of "disability legislation" points out, "without a conception of disability as a social construct" (Liachowitz, 1988, p. 1), an examination of legislation is incomplete.

> What is not accounted for is the fact that laws that deal with handicapped people reflect not only the political problems posed by conflicting interest groups, but also the views that biological deficiency confers social deficiency and that handicapped people deserve (perhaps desire) a place outside of the mainstream of society. Furthermore, useful legislative evaluations need to take into account the processes by which people who deviate from accepted physical norms are devaluated and segregated and, as a result, disabled. (Liachowitz, 1988, p. 1)

As Stone (1984) points out, what a society takes for granted is often much more interesting than its overt controversies. If one removes the contemporary cultural lenses through which disability is normally viewed, the obvious becomes very perplexing indeed" (p. 26). In the following chapter, we turn to these perplexing issues and examine the cultural bases that define disability and set its consequences in each of the nine countries represented at the conference out of which this book grew.

REFERENCES

Becker, H.S. (1963). *Outsiders: Studies in the sociology of deviance.* New York: Free Press.

Bogdan, R., & Taylor, S. J. (1982). *Inside out: The social meaning of mental retardation.* Toronto: University of Toronto Press.

Coles, R. (1979). Introduction. In S. Kleinfield (Ed.), *The hidden minority: A profile of handicapped Americans* (pp. 2–5). Boston: Little, Brown.

Edgerton, R.B. (1970). Mental retardation in non-Western societies: Toward a cross-cultural perspective on incompetence. In H.C. Haywood (Ed.), *Social-cultural aspects of mental retardation* (pp. 523–559). New York: Appleton-Century-Crofts.

Gartner, A., & Joe, T. (Eds.). (1987). *Images of the disabled/disabling images.* New York: Praeger.

Giami, A. (1987). Coping with sexuality of the disabled: A comparison of the physically disabled and the mentally retarded. *International Journal of Rehabilitation Research, 10*(1), 41–48.

Goffman, E. (1963). *Stigma: Notes on the management of spoiled identity.* Englewood Cliffs, NJ: Prentice-Hall.

Goodman, E. (1989). *Making sense.* New York: Atlantic Monthly Press.

Hardy, D. R. (1989, August 21). Social Security's insecure future. *Wall Street Journal,* p. A8.

Haywood, H.C. (1970). *Social-cultural aspects of mental retardation.* New York: Appleton-Century-Crofts.

Liachowitz, C.H. (1988). *Disability as a social construct: Legislative roots.* Philadelphia: University of Pennsylvania Press.

Office of Disability. (1987). *Myths & realities.* Sydney, New South Wales, Australia: Author.

Scott, R.A. (1969). *The making of blind men: A study of adult socialization.* New York: Russell Sage Foundation.

Stone, D.A. (1984). *The disabled state.* Philadelphia: Temple University Press.

APPENDIX

MYTH	REALITY
"Our" people are different.	**People with disabilities have the same needs as non-disabled people. It is the support services which need to be different.**
Assumes that:	Assumes that:
People with disabilities are a separate group to be dealt with differently than others.	People with disabilities are all individuals who can be given opportunities to have their different needs met alongside the rest of the community.
People who run the service know best.	There are plenty of different ways to provide quality services and to involve people with disabilities in decisions about the services they receive.
Some people with disabilities can't make choices.	The effect of some disabilities does make it harder for some people to make choices, but it is never impossible. No-one can make choices unless they have: options from which to choose; understanding and knowledge of what these options are; real experience of different things and the consequences; support to try alternatives.

(continued)

APPENDIX (*continued*)

MYTH	REALITY
The people who have always been in this service don't want it changed.	No-one can make real decisions and choices on the basis of only one experience.
Some people with disabilities can't learn.	All individuals have the capacity to learn.
People with disabilities are "happy" being together.	People with disabilities, like anyone else, may enjoy spending time with people with whom they share common experiences, but it is not usual for this to happen exclusively for the whole of their life.
Any change is for the worse.	Changes based on positive values which promote and support people with disabilities as individual members of society can only be for the better.

MYTH	REALITY
People with disabilities may be able to live in the community only when and if they have achieved certain levels of competency.	**People with disabilities, regardless of disability and their existing level of competency, can and do live, work and participate in the community.**
Assumes that:	Assumes that:
All non-disabled people are competent.	Non-disabled people go on learning and practising new skills throughout their lives.

(continued)

APPENDIX (*continued*)

MYTH	REALITY
People with disabilities learn best in segregated settings.	Just like non-disabled people, people with disabilities learn best in places where they have opportunities to interact with good role models.
The only people who can teach and assist people with disabilities to increase their competence are to be found in larger segregated settings.	There are specialist support workers and services who are assisting people with disabilities to develop, use and practise skills in integrated, community-based settings.
People with intellectual disabilities or challenging behaviours can easily generalise skills from one setting to another.	Some people have difficulty learning skills in one place and then having to practise and use them in another.
People move only when they have received "enough" training (eg, house, work)	People with disabilities should move for the same reasons as the non-disabled population (eg, change of job, new house).
People with disabilities have to earn a place in the community.	People with disabilities do not have to justify that they are members of the community.
The community is not ready and will not accept people who are not as competent as they are.	People in the community do welcome and accept people with disabilities. They do this best when they can get to know people as individuals.
It's the fault of people with disabilities that they	"Blaming the victim" is not a constructive way to

(*continued*)

APPENDIX (*continued*)

MYTH	REALITY
can't do things as well as others.	assist; rather, it's a professional and community challenge to find ways of increasing people's competency and diminishing challenging behaviour.
People with disabilities can't and should not take risks.	An essential part of everyone's learning comes about by having opportunities to take reasonable risks.

MYTH	REALITY
People living in country and outback areas have to depend on one organisation.	**That people who live in outlying areas have the same range of life needs as others and that there are flexible and creative ways of meeting these.**
Assumes that:	Assumes that:
Specialist services are the only ones which can provide services to people with disabilities adequately.	All sorts of agencies and groups available in country or remote areas can provide specialist services with extra resources and training.
People in remote or rural areas have to compromise their individuality because of distance.	Support services which meet individual need can be set up through different service models such as brokerage or coalitions.
One organisation providing all kinds of services is the least restrictive option for	No matter where the location is, one organisation can often provide the most

(continued)

APPENDIX (*continued*)

MYTH	REALITY
people in more isolated areas.	restrictive sorts of services because of the compromises they have to make. Organisations can creatively pursue different ways through negotiating with general agencies, or ensuring different services become autonomous over time.
The first choice for people with disabilities and families in country areas is relocation.	Relocation from one's own home and community should always be the option of last resort. If people continue to consider relocation first then there will be stronger reasons not to create services in the country.

MYTH	REALITY
The principle of "least restrictive alternative" is not applicable to people with severe, profound, or multiple disabilities.	**No matter what the level of support a person requires, they can be provided with services which do not unnecessarily restrict their rights, freedoms, choices, and individual growth and development.**
Assumes that:	Assumes that:
"Least restrictive alternative" is the same as "lesser levels of support".	"Least restrictive alternative" means providing no more and no less support than is required.

(*continued*)

APPENDIX (*continued*)

MYTH	REALITY
People with high levels of support needs don't have the same rights as other people to opportunities that will enhance their independence and competence.	Holding high expectations about all individuals will ensure that people are given opportunities to try new things, experience skills and develop more independence.
People with high levels of support needs will always require the same level of support—this will never change over time.	All people can learn and develop and this will take different techniques, resources or assistance which will vary over time and from time to time.
People with high levels of support needs cannot take risks, live in the community or work.	Others involved in human services are already providing ways for people to live and work in the community.
All those who have more severe disabilities are living in very restrictive and segregated services.	Many individuals with high levels of support needs have always lived in the community.
It is a waste of funds, time and effort to provide services which are the least restrictive.	Having low expectations about individuals results in low achievements.
There are some people who do not have the capacity to achieve outcomes.	The outcomes to which the majority of Australians aspire are those which should apply to all levels of disability. The outcomes remain the same but the way of achieving them will be different for every individual.

(*continued*)

APPENDIX (*continued*)

MYTH	REALITY
	Parents and family members should be involved in decision-making in ways which do not override the needs of the individual with the disability.
The rights of parents/family members are being taken away.	
Assumes that:	Assumes that:
The person with the disability can't make a decision.	People with disabilities can make decisions, and there are ways of helping them do this even if their disability creates problems of understanding and communication.
Parents and family members are the only people who should be involved.	While parents and family members have valuable and unique information and experience, there are others who have specific areas of expertise which are valuable in different ways.
There is no-one else other than the person's family who is interested or wants to be involved.	There are ways of involving other people in the lives of individuals with disabilities so that decisions can be shared by a larger group of concerned people.
Parents and family members have all the information and knowledge on which they can make good decisions.	Parents and family members are often quite unaware of the different kinds of services which may exist and which may be appropriate for their relative.

(continued)

APPENDIX (*continued*)

MYTH	REALITY
Parents are easily able to separate their own needs from those of the person with the disability.	As a result of a lack of family support services, parents often find that their own needs are the same, or more pressing, than those of their son or daughter.
Parents do not want changes to take place for their son or daughter.	Many parents want integrated, community based services and have seen their sons and daughters develop new skills and competencies as a result of these.

Excerpted from Office of Disability.(1978). *Myths & realities*. Sydney, New South Wales, Australia: Author.

2

Culture and Disability

Such are the mysteries of North Korea that diplomats and foreign experts cannot even resolve a basic question about life in Pyongyang: why are there virtually no handicapped people on the capital's broad streets?

[T]he treatment of the handicapped reflects a society's most fundamental values, and in North Korea their absence from the capital appears to reflect the extraordinary enforced orderliness of society. . . .

The suspicion among many foreign residents in North Korea is . . . that President Kim is intensely proud of the capital he built . . . and feels the presence of disabled people would mar the image of the country. (Kristof, 1989, p. A2)

VIEWS OF DISABILITY

Perhaps it is only in a regimented society that one can see cultural values so clearly expressed. In more open societies, some values are expressed obliquely—in the messages contained in advertisements, in the metaphors of everyday speech, as well as in the concepts that underlie public policy. Yet, in either case, cultural and societal values determine people's views on disability.

There is nothing in the nature of disability that makes it the antonym of "orderliness" nor anything that necessarily leads it to "mar" a country's image. These views are interpretations, judgments, and expressions of values.

Responses to impairments are not "natural;" rather they are invented, different at one time or another, from one culture to another. For example, Asch (1988b) cites a recent position paper prepared by the National Association for Sickle Cell Disease. She notes that sickle cell anemia affects one in every 500 black people, making it somewhat more prevalent proportionately than Down syndrome (which affects one in every 800 infants). She says:

> Striking about the position paper is its matter-of-fact treatment of the topic. Its message: part of being black is knowing that a small percentage of individuals carry the gene for the trait and a smaller percentage have the disabling condition. The discussion neither exaggerates nor minimizes the consequences of the condition. . . . Suppose Down syndrome, cystic fibrosis, or spina bifida were depicted not as an incalculable, irreparable tragedy but as a fact of being human? (p. 87)

This was somewhat the case on Martha's Vineyard from the seventeenth through the early part of the twentieth century, when it was the home of the largest concentration of persons who were deaf.

> Most Vineyarders remembered that those who were deaf regarded their inability to hear as a nuisance rather than an overwhelming problem. . . . Most, when pressed on the point, believed that local people, hearing or deaf, preferred to have hearing children, but the birth of a deaf child was regarded as a minor problem rather than a major misfortune. (Groce, 1985, p. 53)

This attitude was a function of the community's inclusion of persons with deafness, particularly through all persons learning sign language, thus addressing the impairment—absence of hearing—and not allowing it to become a handicap. Groce (1985) reinforces the point, noting:

> Only two deaf men were considered to be handicapped, according to the Islanders. The first, a farmer and fisherman, had lost his right hand in a mowing machine accident as a teenager, and hence was said to be handicapped. . . . The other handicapped deaf individual apparently had difficulty walking. (pp. 127–128)

Although we can categorize the deaf Vineyarders as disabled, they certainly were not considered to be handicapped. They participated freely in all aspects of life in this Yankee community. They grew up, married, raised their families, and earned their living in just the same manner as did their hearing relatives, friends, and neighbors.

Perhaps the best description of the status of deaf individuals on the Vineyard was given . . . by an island woman in her eighties, when . . . asked about those who were handicapped by deafness when she was a girl: "Oh," she said emphatically, "those people weren't handicapped. They were just deaf." (p. 4–5)

Kenneth Jernigan (1985), in his presidential address at the annual convention of the National Federation of the Blind, made a similar point:

Sight is enjoyable; it is convenient. But that is all that it is— enjoyable, useful, convenient. Except in imagination and mythology it is not the single key to human happiness, the road to knowledge, or the window to the soul. Like the other senses, it is a channel of communication, a source of pleasure, and a tool— nothing less, nothing more. It is alternative, not exclusive. It is certainly not the essential component of human freedom. (p. 387)

In a study of the new techniques of reproductive technology, Rapp (1988) interviewed parents of children with disabilities and found:

Families whose children have the same conditions that amniocentesis now diagnoses prenatally speak counterdiscourses to medical authority. Here, religion, ethnicity, class and family history powerfully shape responses to having a child with a genetically stigmatized condition. Reflections on the meaning of maternity and paternity and the value of children are embedded in the stories parents of the disabled [sic] tell as they transform medical diagnosis into the social fabric of daily life. Strategies for coping and making cultural meaning through a life crisis and family transformation vary enormously. (p. 112)

Echoing Asch's point, above, a black mother of a child with Down syndrome says, "My kid's got a heart problem, my kid's gonna be slow. First let me deal with that, love him for that, then I'll check out this Down Syndrome thing" (cited in Rapp, 1988, p. 112).

Culture affects how others view disability and treat persons with disabilities, and it affects the individuals themselves. Bogdan (1980) interviewed persons who had been labeled "retarded," who nonetheless said, "I'm not retarded." He quotes one of them, who says, "I have never really thought of myself as

retarded. I never really had that ugly feeling deep down" (p. 76).
Biklen (n.d.) expands on this self-perception:

> The largest single self advocacy organization of people labelled as
> retarded calls itself "People First". Marsha Saxton, a person with
> Spina Bifida reports, "As I see it, I'm not lucky or unlucky. I'm just
> the way I am. But I'm not disabled, I always thought. Or handi-
> capped" (Saxton, 1985, p. 129). Denise Karuth, who also has a
> physical disability, sounds like a modern day Win [in Margaret
> Kennedy's novel, *Not in the Calendar*] when she writes, "Put your
> handkerchiefs away. I'm a lot more like you than you possibly
> imagine" (Karuth, 1985, p. 12). The message in each of these
> instances . . . is that a disability is only one dimension of a per-
> son, not all-defining and not inherently a barrier to being recog-
> nized as fully human. (p. 7)

Kuhn's (1962) concept of a paradigm, namely the way in
which one views (or organizes) a body of information, expresses
the idea of a conceptual model or map that is used to make sense
of things. It is not the phenomena that change but rather the
way(s) of ordering, understanding, and responding to them. For
example, Mercer (1988) points out that in the United States
what she calls the "IQ paradigm" is being replaced by a new way
of understanding knowledge. One of the consequences of this,
she says, is that the whole apparatus of categorizing children
based upon IQ scores and the service system of education (special and general) that has grown up around this apparatus
necessarily will change. Among other things this will produce
changes in the conduct of education; the operation of schools;
and the utilization of personnel, their preparation, and rewards.

The point for us, then, is that the way in which something
is understood—the cultural meaning—has consequence not
only as a matter of understanding but also for actions that are
based upon or grow out of that understanding.[1] In Chapters 4
through 9, we examine practices based upon differing national
understandings of disability. In the remainder of this chapter,
we look at some of these different ways of understanding dis-

---

[1]An interesting new book (Tobin, Wu, & Davidson, 1989) examines preschool in three cultures (China, Japan, and the United States) and notes that
the ways in which such programs are conceptualized and designed is a function of basic societal factors, for example, "the egalitarian thrust of the Com-
munist revolution in China, the post-occupation, democratic educational-re-
form movement in Japan, and, in the United States, the twentieth century
diffusion of the middle-class dream of upward social mobility through education. . ." (p. 26).

ability. In doing this, we are mindful of the caution expressed by Langness (1987):

> That all theories of behavior, society, culture and evolution were based upon the behavior of western Europeans [and their colonial progeny] or on biased accounts of other people is a fact of great significance in the history of science and should not be ignored. (p. 201)

CULTURAL JUDGMENTS REGARDING DISABILITY

The phrase "impairment as a human constant" is both the title of a useful survey article (Scheer & Groce, 1988) and the expression of a simple reality. Summarizing the data from prehistoric evidence, Scheer and Groce (1988) found, "Virtually every reported large skeletal population includes at least one individual, and often several, whose remains show congenital malformations, improperly healed bones, missing limbs, or head trauma" (p. 27). Yet, "anthropologists and sociologists have usually dismissed the disabled individuals they have encountered as liminal figures, temporary anomalies in a non-handicapped population" (Groce, 1985, p. 108).

What varies, the authors state, is how over the course of history "societies have defined what did and did not constitute a disability or a handicap" (Scheer & Groce, 1988, p. 23). For example, while among the Incas persons with disabilities were sent outside of the city on fiesta days (Rowe, 1946), Mead (1928) reports that in Samoa persons with physical disabilities were included in ceremonial dancing.

Turning to the place of persons with disabilities in traditional societies, historic and present-day, Scheer & Groce (1988) suggest that biases among Western social scientists about the marginal human nature of persons with disabilities have affected understanding. So, too, has cultural chauvinism. The author of an anthropology textbook wrote, "Biologically handicapped children are a humanistic concern in our society, whereas in simple human populations they died early and were not missed" (Birdsell, 1972, p. 384).

Again challenging the accepted wisdom, Scheer and Groce (1988) report that a number of common beliefs do not stand up to scrutiny: "A careful review of the ethnographic literature reveals no reports of societies in which disabled people are routinely put to death if they survive past infancy, or become disabled later in their lives" (p. 27), and "The belief . . . that disabled persons in traditional societies usually occupy the role of shaman, priest, or priestess is suspect" (p. 28).

Where infanticide against persons with disabilities does occur, Scheer and Groce (1988) note that the most common justification "is the belief that they represent an evil spirit, perhaps the off-spring of a human mother and a supernatural being" (p. 28). Pointing out that "the belief in the linkage between evil spirits and/or parental misconduct and the birth of a disabled newborn appears widespread," present in both earlier, nonindustrial as well as in contemporary, industrial societies, they state, "In societies that view one's present state as a reflection of past misdeeds and transgressions, the life of a disabled child or adult may be made difficult, with sharply limited social and economic options" (p. 28). For example, in many religions, such as Shinto and Buddhism, "disabled people [are viewed] as a curse on the family. They [are] seen as badges of shame which indicated that the family might have committed some sin in the past" (Driedger, 1989, p. 16).

Florian (1987), in analyzing the dimensions of culture in attitudes toward disability, contrasts shame-oriented versus guilt-oriented cultures. "Shame and guilt", he says, "differ from other affects in that they may be understood through their direct references to internalized social norms: the disruption or violation of these social norms may lead to 'shame'—a response to role transgression—or 'guilt'—a response to moral transgression" (p. 41).

> In a "shame-oriented" society most individuals' reactions to a stigmatizing condition, such as a physical disability, may involve attempts to hide the condition from the immediate surroundings, while in a "guilt-oriented" society individuals' reactions to such a condition may involve ongoing self-blame and a strong sense of personal responsibility for the condition. Shame interrupts, exposes and disrupts a unitary sense of an individual and his/her family, while guilt evaluates, judges and condemns the individual and his/her family. (pp. 41–42)

And, while persons with disabilities are not universally assigned a particular role, such as that of priest, "in many preindustrial and some industrial societies, begging is a traditional role for [those, including persons with disabilities] who find themselves without the protection of kin and community social alliances. Throughout the Moslem world, for example, giving alms to the disabled is a social obligation" (p. 29). And, Miles (1983) points out:

> Dropping coins into the blind beggar's bowl may lead to avoidance of punishment in the afterlife. . . . The disabled beggar asks for "justice". Since fate, Karma, or deity has deprived him [sic], begging becomes his rightful duty and occupation: justice demands that his bowl be filled. If the unseen forces present a poor family with a deformed baby, it is the family's duty to exploit the deformity for financial gain. (p. 27)

As noted in Chapter 1, the definition of disabled—and thus, according to Miles, of those entitled to beg—is not a simple or straightforward matter. Indeed, as Stone (1984) points out:

> There are published stories from as far back as the fifth century B.C. to the effect that people feigned madness to avoid military service or other obligations. In English reports and laws of the fifteenth through nineteenth century, there are innumerable descriptions of beggars' schemes for pretending to be crippled and blind, artfully producing counterfeit sores, lacerating themselves, and feigning epileptic fits, pregnancy, dropsy, or leprosy. In France, one particular order of beggars, the *mitoux*, were allegedly trained in medicine so that they could "produce the appearance of every kind of malady and even deceive doctors themselves." (p. 32)

In fact, Stone (1984) argues that while the two other categories of contemporary social welfare policy, that is, childhood and old age, are assumed to represent authentic states of being, totally independent of the will of individuals,

> disability, on the other hand, even in its early incarnations as more specific conditions, was seen to exist in both genuine and artificial forms. People could either be truly injured or feign injury. In the modern understanding of disability, deception has become part and parcel of the concept itself, and the nature of this deception is tied to the particular form of validation used to detect it. The definition of disability and the means to determine it became critically linked. (p. 28)

In a unique[2] description of persons with onchocercous blindness in the small Mexican village of San Pedro Yolox, Gwaltney (1970) describes "the role of mendicancy in the maintenance of a sense of participation [in the life of the community] on the part of the blind. . ." (pp. v–vi). Accommodative adjustment to blindness is expressed by

> the transgenerational link between the elderly onchocercous blind and child guides, ... the ascription of ritual efficacy and public merit to deferential behavior toward blind persons, and the obverse ascription of strong supernatural and social opprobrium to undeferential behavior toward them, and the absence of curative traits from indigenous medical technology and sorcery. . . . (Gwaltney, 1970, pp. v–vi)

While in some cultures, as Scheer and Groce have noted, persons with disabilities are seen as representing an evil spirit, in San Pedro Yolox there is "the widespread belief that the blind are under special divine protection. . ." (Gwaltney, 1970, p. 111). This appears to be the source of the deference given to them and the children's desire to serve them,[3] as well as the belief that they are "protected against the bite of venomous snakes and the shock of lightning" (Gwaltney, 1970, p. 111). But more important than belief in supernatural protection is the assistance provided by family members and other villagers. This also is true for those with the same condition in West Africa, where the condition is called "river blindness." "Blind people can often be absorbed into the extended family. Indeed, some can even prosper. In one village . . . the chief, resplendent in white robes, had kept his power and prestige through 18 years of blindness" (Eckholm, 1989, p. 25).

In the following sections, we illustrate differences in cultural roles by looking at two groups among persons with disabilities—persons with deafness and women with disabilities.

---

[2]The study is made particularly interesting by the fact that the author is himself blind and a black man, who was in the village during the time of the assaults on black people in Montgomery. In their welcome to him, the village elders said, "We are a poor people and many of us do not have much education, but we have the natural wisdom which God gives even the humblest of His children. So there is no one among us who would demean himself by abusing another human being simply because his skin is darker" (Gwaltney, 1970, pp. 2–3).

[3]The author's use of a cane for mobility was strange to the villagers and the children were quite insistent upon wanting to "guide" him, an offer he accepted in light of the rocky and hilly terrain of the village (Gwaltney, 1970, pp. 113–114).

Persons with Deafness

Just as the role of persons with blindness has varied over time and culture, so too has the role of persons with deafness. Groce (1985) uses a relevant summary as a framework for her study of Martha's Vineyard (pp. 98–105). While early Babylonian laws restricted the rights of persons born deaf, the Mosaic Code (sixth century B.C.) warned against cursing deaf persons. Four hundred years later, Talmudic rabbis included persons with congenital deafness in the same category as children and those with mental retardation and endorsed laws that restricted them from the legal rights and responsibilities of other citizens.

The ideas of Aristotle and his contemporaries had the most far reaching implications. Given their belief that speech was the medium of thought and education, those who could not hear were seen as incapable of learning. This view came to be incorporated in Roman science. Lucretius wrote, "To instruct the deaf no art could reach/ No care improve them, and no wisdom teach" (cited in Burnet, 1835, cited in Groce, 1985, p. 53).

The Justinian Code (6th century A.D.) made a sharp distinction between those who were born with deafness and those who lost their hearing after having acquired language.[4] The legal rights of the former were sharply curtailed; and, perhaps more consequentially, in the Middle Ages, they were seen as incapable of having religious faith. St. Augustine wrote, "deafness from birth makes faith impossible, since he who is born deaf can neither hear the word nor learn it" (Seiss, 1887, cited in Groce,

---

[4]A critical question, of course, is what is identified as "language?" "In hearing people's milieu, languages are spoken; since deaf people rarely speak, hearing professionals have long concluded that deaf people have no language at their command" (Lane, 1988, p. 10). A contrary view sees American Sign Language (or its equivalents in other countries) as "the equal of English as a natural language. . ." (Lane, 1988, p. 9).

[5]Assertions of the relationship between impairment and capacity to develop are not limited to the now discredited views of Aristotle and St. Augustine. For example, Gliedman and Roth (1980) point out that in order to apply Erikson's typology of human development to persons with disabilities, we must "approach disability by means of a deviance analysis, looking at the problems of the handicapped by identifying specific areas of potential deviance for each stage." They say that this requires one to "prejudge precisely those developmental questions about handicap which, above all others, require painstaking empirical investigation. . ." (p. 106). They indicate that a further issue concerns

1985, p. 155).[5] This view was incorporated into medieval systems of law, so that in many places persons born deaf were not permitted to marry, have a voice in government, or inherit property.

During the era of Enlightenment, there were a number of instances of education of children with deafness whose families were wealthy. "The instructors often were prompted as much by intellectual curiosity as by compassion for the children" (Groce, 1985, p. 100). By the middle of the seventeenth century, there were increasing efforts to consider education for children with deafness. The circumstances were hardly favorable, the author of the first English treatise on deaf education, John Bulwer, wrote, "The condition that they are in who are born deafe and dumbe, is indeed very sad and lamentable: for they are looked upon as misprisions in nature, and wanting speech are reckoned little better than Dumbe Animals" (Bulwer, 1648, p. 102).[6]

In the course of the eighteenth century, schools for persons with deafness were established in Paris, Leipzig, and Edin-

---

the typology's incorporation at each higher stage of the most salient features of the lower stages. Thus, for example, the child's mastery of bodily functions, which is central to resolving the second stage's issues of autonomy versus shame and doubt, remains an open issue for the adult person with a disability who either lacks bladder control or is dependent upon an attendant (or a family member). Thus, "there is an 'infantile' quality to the way he [sic] must assert his mastery over his body. Like the young child who must call on his mother [sic] for help, the physically handicapped person must sometimes relate to his own body by means of another (able-bodied) person" (p. 107). While this aspect of the typology suggests that persons with disabilities cannot move on to the higher stages of development, Gliedman and Roth also point out that the typology does not well address the great precocity that many persons with disabilities display in their interpersonal behavior. They conclude that one cannot approach the development of a child with disabilities "on terms spelled out in advance by personality theories developed for able-bodied children and adults" (p. 113). This approach would lead to no more accurate data about them than has the development of stages of moral growth drawing solely from data concerning males. As Gilligan (1979) has pointed out, women have been missing even as subjects in the research about psychological development. In words that are exactly analogous to our concerns here, Belenky, Clinchy, Goldberger, and Tarule (1986) write, "This omission of women from scientific studies is almost universally ignored when scientists draw conclusions from their findings and generalize what they have learned from the study of men to lives of women" (p. 6).

[6]In a trenchant comment on the distance between traditional scholarship and the reality of everyday life, Groce (1985) notes that at the same time as this was written, on Martha's Vineyard persons with deafness were living as full participants in community life, presumably communicating with other community members, deaf and hearing alike, through sign language.

burgh, although the Abbé de l'Epée, who founded what later was to become the National Institute for Deaf Mutes, found that "very respectable ecclesiastics . . . openly condemned deaf education for theological reasons" (Mann, 1836, p. 103). While the establishment of such schools, as well as many others in the course of the nineteenth century in Western Europe and North America, led to improvements in the lives of those persons with deafness who attended them, they only served to heighten the disdain in which persons with deafness were held. A nineteenth century American scholar complained that some believed "that deaf mutes, left to themselves, would rise no higher than orang-outangs. . ." (Jenkins, 1890, p. 185).

Key to the inclusion of persons with deafness in the community of Martha's Vineyard was the widespread use of sign language.[7] It was the tool of accessibility. As Groce (1985) reports:

> It was not simply a question of language usage; the attitude of hearing people toward the deaf and their ability to communicate easily and well extended into every aspect of Vineyard society. There was no language barrier and, by extension, there seems to have been no social barrier. (p. 75)

> The social aspects of day-to-day life on the Vineyard provide a feeling of what life was like for the deaf in these communities. Hearing and deaf people intermingled everywhere—at home, at the general store, at church, at parties. Participation by deaf family, friends, and neighbors was a normal part of everyday life. (p. 87)

> As with all other aspects of Island life, in socializing no one made any distinctions between deaf people and hearing people. No one was able to give me an example of social activities in which only the deaf participated. Unlike the mainland, where various deaf clubs and activities are the center of social interaction for many deaf people, the Vineyard activities were attended by the deaf and the hearing. It was not simply that the hearing Islanders welcomed the deaf into their midst; the deaf Islanders apparently made no attempt to set up activities independent of their hearing family, friends, and neighbors. If a deaf Islander wanted to entertain only other deaf individuals, he or she probably would have had to exclude spouse, siblings, children, best friends, or immediate neighbors, all of whom would have been hurt. (p. 93)

---

[7]There is considerable dispute as to the nature of the deaf community and the appropriate setting for the education of youngsters with deafness. However, there is agreement as to the absence of spoken language as the key factor in the isolation of persons with deafness from the broader community.

And, in a turnabout, sign language was used between hearing people. Groce (1985) reports that parents who did not want young children to "hear" their conversation spoke in sign! She cites a 1885 newspaper story reporting on housewives on farms wide distances from each other conversing in sign using a spyglass to see each other. And "Sign language was used by fishermen in boats on the open water. One man recalled, 'Fishermen hauling [lobster] pots . . . would discuss how the luck was running. . . . These men could talk and hear alright, but it'd be too far to yell'" (p. 65).

While in some cultures persons with disabilities were seen as representing an evil spirit, many other explanations for disability have been proffered. For example:

> Over the years numerous reasons for [Martha's] Vineyard deafness were put forward: the will of God, the sins of the father, fright during pregnancy. Alexander Graham Bell,[8] who visited the Island and wrote several papers on it, thought the deafness might be caused by the layer of clay under the soil of Chilmark but not of the other towns of the Vineyard, where deafness was less common. (Groce, 1985, p. viii)

Women with Disabilities

The power of social conditions is seen most explicitly in examining the status of women with disabilities, who are "trapped in two socially devalued roles. . ." (Fine & Asch, 1985, p. 13). Attention to women with disabilities, what Deegan and Brooks (1985) have called "the double handicap,"[9] has grown in the past several years, sparked by Fine and Asch's (1985) essay, "Disabled women: sexism without the pedestal." (See in particular, four collections of essays: Browne, Connors, & Stern, 1985; Deegan & Brooks, 1985; Fine & Asch, 1989.)

Fine and Asch (1985) note that women with disabilities are viewed more negatively than men with disabilities, both in self-

---

[8]Bell, an advocate of immigration restriction and eugenics, warned of the possible "Formation of a deaf variety of the Human Race" (1883) and advocated measures to disperse the deaf community (Longmore, 1987, p. 357).

[9]A further multiplication of the situation occurs in the instance of Sharon Kowalski. At issue, in a protracted conflict between the woman's parents and her lesbian partner, is who will make decisions about treatment (Ms. Kowalkski was severely injured by a drunken driver) and living arrangements (Brozan, 1988, p. 28).

perceptions and the perceptions of others. They not only are more likely to internalize society's rejection, but, furthermore, they are also more likely than men with disabilities to identify themselves as "disabled." This is true for both those who are born with a disability, as well as those who acquire a disability later. Indeed, they point out that "disability carries with it such a powerful imputation of inability to perform any adult social function[10] that there is no other descriptor needed by the public" (p. 12). Historically, persons with disabilities who have achieved greatly, such as Beethoven, Milton, Julius Caesar, and in our own time Franklin Delano Roosevelt, are not viewed as persons who had disabilities. Gallagher (1985), in a unique biography of Roosevelt, *FDR's Splendid Deception*, points out that only two out of 35,000 Hyde Park Library photographs show him in a wheelchair, and, said the wife of a former Roosevelt advisor, "we never, ever thought of the President as handicapped, we never thought of it at all" (p. 210). In commenting on this, Longmore (1987) says, "Surely she did not mean that they were oblivious to his physical condition. Rather, she and probably most Americans exempted FDR from the dependent social role and the devalued social identity imposed on people with disabilities" (pp. 360–361).

Kent (1987) describes her attempts as a young woman with blindness to find role models in literature "for the woman I might some day hope to become" (p. 47). In an essay surveying a range of books, she concludes:

> Disability sets the tone for the woman's interactions with others. Her competence at homemaking chores, her educational attainments, or her personality have little effect upon the attitudes of others toward her. As other characters react to her disability they are not concerned about her competence, but something much deeper and harder to define. Disability seems to undermine the very roots of her womanhood. (p. 63)

This devaluation occurs not only in the United States. Speaking of women with disabilities in the Third World, a Pakistani doctor with a visual impairment wrote:

---

[10]An aspect of this is documented by Giami (1987) who notes that the professional literature about the sexual lives of persons with paraplegia "is mostly (almost always) concerned with paraplegic men and able-bodied women. The question of maintenance of relations and the 'reconquest' of the able-bodied partner in the case of paraplegic women is rarely dealt with" (p. 44).

Women in general have power as wives and mothers within the home, and their status in society comes from this role. A disabled woman, in general, cannot share in this status. She is not seen as *marriageable* [italics in the original]—no one wants to arrange a marriage with "damaged goods." Also, in the developing world, women perform most of the labor in the home and on the fields. A disabled woman often cannot perform this work as efficiently as a nondisabled woman. Consequently a disabled woman has no status because she cannot accomplish those tasks which bring women status in her society. (cited in Driedger, 1989, p. 16)

HIERARCHIES OF DEVELOPMENT

In a landmark monograph examining mental retardation in non-Western societies, Edgerton (1970) points to a common fallacy.

Complex societies produce many difficulties for the retarded, whereas simpler societies can absorb such persons as useful, even productive, members. This, then is the conventional, cultural relativistic understanding in a nutshell: Complex, industrial societies demand greater intellectual competence than do small, technologically simple societies. In vulgar terms, the understanding reads as follows: Simple people for simple societies. (p. 525)

Hanks and Hanks (1948) have put forward, in a nonvulgar fashion, such a concept. They suggest

that individuals who are disabled have more social participation and physical protection in small-scale, relatively egalitarian societies, where group cooperation takes precedence over competition and productivity is much the same for all members. (Groce, 1985, p. 107)

Challenging this argument, Groce (1985) points out that Martha's Vineyard was in no stretch of the imagination an egalitarian society where cooperation was more important than competition.

Vineyarders, hearing and deaf, were responsible for supporting themselves and their families. Paying bills, mortgages and taxes; selling the harvest or catching fish, running for office, holding a town post or participating in old-fashioned Yankee horse trading—all these responsibilities placed deaf Vineyarders squarely in the modern competitive world. Some grew wealthy, most got by, and a few simply scraped by, just as the hearing members of their families did. (pp. 107–108)

These dichotomous views exist in a line of thinking regarding the conceptualizations of intelligence and development of "higher" and "lower" levels of thinking: "'concrete' modes of thought which are 'lower' than 'abstract' modes of thought, prelogical as opposed to logical modes, animistic as opposed to scientific modes, and the like" (Langness, 1987, p. 41).

Giami (1987) illustrates an aspect of this thinking in a discussion of attitudes about sexuality among persons with mental retardation.

> Those professionally involved in special education [in France] have a conception in which the sexuality of the mentally retarded may be described as 'primitive' and incomplete in relation to the genital model. It is primitive in that educators highlight the most visible and provocative elements of that sexuality. They report individual and collective masturbatory activity, exhibitionism, and voyeurism, and aggressive and homosexual behaviour. Such practices are depicted as irrepressible and devoid of emotion. Lastly, the mentally retarded are presented as incapable of having full sexual relations. (p. 46)

Such hierarchies make sense, of course, only in the context of some form of arbitrarily imposed and culture-bound metric. "The decision to classify one task as somehow higher than another is fundamentally an arbitrary one, and it is relative to the culture in which the decision is made" (Langness, 1987, p. 42).

> Every culture has its myths. One of our most persistent is that nonliterate people in less developed countries possess something we like to call a 'primitive mentality' that is both different from and inferior to our own. This myth has it that the 'primitive mind' is highly concrete, whereas the 'Western mind' is highly abstract; the 'primitive mind' connects its concrete ideas by rote associations, whereas the 'Western mind' connects its abstract ideas by general relations; the 'primitive mind' is illogical and insensitive to contradictions, while the 'Western mind' is logical and strives to attain consistency; the 'primitive mind' is childish and emotional, whereas the 'Western mind' is mature and rationale; and so on and so on. (Miller, 1971, p. ii)

Gardner's (1983) concept of multiple intelligences is an effort to break out of such arbitrary bounds.[11] He defines intelligence as the ability to solve a problem or to fashion a product in a way that is considered useful in one or more cultural set-

---

[11]For his application of the multiple intelligences concept to the evaluation and education of students now labeled handicapped, see Goldman and Gardner (1989).

tings. In this regard, intelligence comes to be understood as contextual rather than hierarchical. An example of this is found in the work of Michael Cole and his colleagues (Cole, Gay, Glick, & Sharp, 1971), who "found that the Kpelle of Liberia, who appear to be inferior to Europeans in mathematics and memory, can perform as well as Europeans or even better when the experiments used to test these skills are appropriate to Kpelle culture" (Edgerton & Langness, 1974, p. 100).

The hierarchical or evolutionary concepts extend to ways of thinking in various fields, indeed across fields, linking the stages of human development to stages of the development of societies. Freud was familiar with the theories of the evolutionists, incorporating their concepts into his work:

> The era to which the dream-work takes us back is 'primitive' in a two-fold sense: in the first place, it means the early days of the individual—his [sic] childhood—and secondly, in so far as each individual repeats in some abbreviated fashion during childhood the whole course of the development of the human race, the reference is phylogenetic. (Freud, 1920, p. 177, cited in Langness, 1987, p. 39)

Jung carried this idea even further:

> All this experience suggests to us that we draw the parallel between the phantastical, mythological thinking of antiquity and the similar thinking of children, between the lower human races and dreams. . . . [T]he state of infantile thinking in the child's psychic life, as well as in dreams, is nothing but a re-echo of the prehistoric and ancient. (Jung, 1916, pp. 27–28 cited in Langness, 1987, p. 40)

And in the field of medicine, along these same lines, Dr. J. Langdon H. Down wrote in 1866:

> I have for some time had my attention directed to the possibility of making a classification of the feeble-minded by arranging them around various ethnic standards. . . . [T]he great Mongolian family has numerous representatives, and it is to this division, I wish to call special attention. A very large number of congenital idiots are typical Mongols. So marked is this, that when placed side by side, it is difficult to believe the specimens compared are not children of the same parents. (Langness, 1987, pp. 46–47)

Down goes on to describe one such young man, and concludes, "The boy's aspect is such that it is difficult to realize that he is the child of Europeans, but so frequently are these characteristics presented, that there can be no doubt that these ethnic features are the result of degeneration" (Langness, 1987, p. 47). In medical terms, this idea of degeneration can be formulated with health being seen as an evolution, disease as a dissolution. In this view, "the mentally diseased person is a sane man [sic] who has been pushed down a few steps in evolution" (Van den Berg, 1961, p. 64, cited in Langness, 1987). Langness (1987) notes the commonplace reference to persons with retardation as childlike and those with mental illness as "savages." Thus, the equation: primitives = ethnic minorities = children = persons with mental retardation = persons with mental illness, and so forth.

A similarly negative point of view was expressed in a doctor's 1895 explanation of deafness on Martha's Vineyard.

> There is a secluded hamlet on the Island of Martha's Vineyard called Chilmarth [sic]. This community, isolated from the outer, larger, pulsing world, has not only retained its primitive customs and manners, but the physical taint in the original stock has also produced a plenteous harvest of affliction. (S. Millington Miller, cited in Groce, 1985, p. 94).

And professional journals were not free of this view. An 1858 article in the *American Annals of the Deaf and Dumb* stated:

> Before going through a course of instructional discipline, the deaf and dumb are guided almost wholly by instinct and their animal passion. They have no more opportunity of cultivating the intellect and reasoning faculties than the savages of Patagonia or the North American Indians. (cited in Groce, 1985, p. 102)

Similar stereotypes are present in today's professional writing. From the *Journal of the American Academy of Child Psychiatry:* "Suspiciousness . . . as well as impulsiveness and aggressive behaviors have been reported as typical of deaf adults. [R]ecent reports have tended to confirm these judgments" (cited in Lane, 1988, p. 7). And from a widely cited survey of the literature on the "psychology of the deaf," "rigidity, emotional immaturity, [and] social ineptness" are cited as predominant characteristics (cited in Lane, 1988, p. 7).

Going beyond a critique of the stereotypic characterizations of persons with deafness, Lane (1988) states:

There is no psychology of the deaf. It is, in fact, not clear that there *can* [italics in the original] be one. The term may inevitably represent the pathologizing of cultural differences, the interpretation of difference as deviance. (p. 16)

The consideration of persons with disabilities as if they were a "primitive" group is strikingly illustrated by Lane (1988), who presents a comparison of the traits attributed to African people in the literature of colonialism, which reflects its narrowmindedness and arrogance (Table 2.1) and those attributed to people with deafness in the professional literature (Table 2.2).

As Lane (1988) points out, "the list of traits attributed to deaf people is inconsistent. . . . The list is, however, consistently negative" (p. 8). In both cases, this inconsistency of trait attributions and their negativity, Lane says, "may reveal little about Africans or deaf people, but much about the colonial authorities or hearing authorities and the social contexts in which they operate" (p. 8). It is, Lane asserts, a system of paternalistic stereotypes, one in which those in control—that is those doing the attribution—seek to gain control over the as-

Table 2.1.   Some traits attributed to African people in the literature of colonialism

Social	Cognitive	Behavioral	Emotional
Barbaric	No arts	Alcoholic	Carefree
Bloodthirsty	No business	Animalistic	Emotional
Cannibalistic	Cunning	Childlike	Excitable
Coarse	Fast learners	Diligent	Fatalistic
No conscience	Frivolous	Dirty	Fickle
Cruel	Ignorant	Feeble	Fierce
Depraved	Improvident	Ill-fed	Hilarious
Discouraged	Insolent	Impulsive	Passive
No economy	Intelligent	Lazy	Proud
Gregarious	Irrational	Orgiastic	
Secretive	Mentally lazy	Restrained	Servile
Submissive			
Treacherous	Suspicious	Shy	Vengeful
Unrepentant	Unimaginative	Stunted	
Unstable	Unintelligent	Superficial	

(Adapted from Lane [1988], p. 8.)

Table 2.2. Some traits attributed to deaf people in the professional literature

Social	Cognitive	Behavioral	Emotional
Admiration (depends on)	Conceptual thinking poor	Aggressive	Anxiety (lack of)
Asocial	Concrete	Androgynous	Depressive
Clannish	Doubting	Conscientious	Emotionally disturbed
Competitive	Egocentric	Hedonistic	Emotionally immature
Conscience weak	Failure externalized	Immature	Empathy (lack of)
Credulous	Failure internalized	Impulsive	Explosive
Dependent	Insight poor	Initiative lacking	Frustrated easily
Disobedient	No introspection	Interests few	Irritable
Immature	No language	Motor development slow	Moody
Irresponsible	Language poor	Personality undeveloped	Neurotic
Role rigid	Mechanically inept	Possessive	Paranoid
Shy	Naive	Rigid	Passionate
Socially undeveloped	Reasoning restricted	Shuffling gait	Psychotic reactions
Submissive	Self-awareness poor	Stubborn	Serious
Suggestible	Shrewd	Suspicious	Temperamental
Unsocialized	Thinking unclear	Unconfident	Unfeeling
	Unaware		
	Unintelligent		

(Adapted from Lane [1988], p. 9.)

cribed. Lane's broader views about persons with deafness (1984) are beyond the scope of our concern here; the point we wish to emphasize in this treatment of culture and disability is the similarity between the ways persons viewed as "primitive" and persons with disabilities are portrayed.

Given the data as to the differential roles that persons with impairments play in Western and non-Western societies, rather than a simplistic, environmental, and mechanistic determinism, Edgerton (1970) suggests that one must look to the "web that unites culture and social organizations within their physical environment" (p. 547). Scheer and Groce (1988) do just that.

> In small-scale societies . . . regular face-to-face contact between community members is frequent. Individuals are related and connected to each other in diffuse social roles and contexts. In such situations, a single personal characteristic, such as a physical impairment, does not generalize to define one's total social identity. In complex societies, however, social relationships and contexts are more impersonal and task specific, and individuals are not related to each other in varied contexts. Accordingly, visible physical characteristics are commonly used to classify and socially notate the individual's identity. (p. 32f.)

Alden Nowlan's poem, "He's lived there all his life" (cited in Biklen, 1989), describing the treatment of a person with blindness, illustrates both of Scheer's and Groce's points.

> Nowlan writes of a blind man who receives differential treatment from the "locals" of the small town and its "newcomers." The "newcomers" treat the man with a measure of charity, even patronizingly. The manager of the local movie theatre gives the man a ride to the movies when a new show opens. Others read him the newspapers. Some listen patiently to the man's boring stories. . . . Newcomers feel sorry for the "poor old man" whom they say the locals treat badly. Nowlan sides with the locals, observing that in a small town people can come to know each other so well that a person's lack of sight does not cloud people's appreciation or disdain for each others' behavior. (p. 235)

LITERARY IMAGES OF PERSONS WITH DISABILITIES

The examination of literature to understand the images it portrays of persons with disabilities is growing (among many works, see especially Fiedler, 1984; Kent, 1987, 1989; Kriegel, 1987; Sontag, 1979). Zola (1985) summarizes the treatment of persons with disabilities according to several recurring themes: feelings of pity and fear; menace and loathing; perceptions of innocence (e.g., the eternal child); wonderment ("super crip"); and a view of people as victims, indicated by the use of terms such as "victims of" and "sufferers of" (p. 5). Biklen (n.d.), in seeking the analogues in public policy of the images of persons with disabilities in literature, identified portrayals of persons with disabilities as: different, untouchable, charity's burden, burdensome to other people, offensive, in need of being managed, an impediment to the freedom of others, the patients, dangerous, unacceptable, and trapped.

Kriegel (1987) describes literature's "demonic cripple" (e.g., Shakespeare's King Richard and Melville's Ahab); the "charity cripple" (e.g., Dickens's Tiny Tim); the "realistic cripple" (e.g., William's Laura); the "survivor cripple" (e.g., Bellow's William Einhorn). Of course, the view of the world—including the world of persons with disabilities—that produces these images is not from the disabled person's perspective;[12] "most writers look at the cripple [sic] and the wounds he [sic] bears with the same suspicion and distaste that are found in other 'normals'" (Kriegel, 1987, p. 33). Furthermore:

> The cripple is the creature who has been deprived of his ability to create a self. If others cry, like God from the burning bush, "I am that I am," the cripple in literature is expected to submit to the cries of others to say, "I am what you tell me I am." He is the other, if for no other reason than that only by being the other will he be allowed to presume upon the society of the "normals". He must accept definition from outside the boundaries of his own existence. (pp. 33–34)

Kent (1987, 1989) expands Kriegel's analysis from men with physical disabilities to women with blindness. She reports that blind characters in literature were either "living in a terrifying death-like world of darkness, being punished for past sins (often sexual in nature) and to be feared" or possessed "superhuman powers and insights" and were "morally superior" to sighted people (cited in Johnson, 1989b, p. 9). In either case, they were not real characters as much as symbols. The same was found to be true in a study by two Gallaudet professors about characters with deafness; that is, they were not realistic but either demonized or, more usually, idealized (Johnson, 1989b, p. 10):

> What's absent in these accounts is reality—the sense that disabled people are normal human beings up against a flawed sys-

---

[12]The extent to which this is the case is illustrated by a report (Solomon, 1987) that Douglas Bullard's novel, *Islay*, is the first published novel about the "deaf experience" written by a person with deafness.

tem. It's easier to pretend disabled people are essentially different than to focus on the social conditions we've set up that have caused them to live in abnormal ways. (Johnson, 1989b, p. 10)

SOCIAL RESOURCES

The Poor Laws of late sixteenth century England included persons with physical disabilities among other "defectives" and "vagrants" who were granted community protection (Stone, 1984). They were distinguished from the nondisabled and "unworthy" poor who were seen as malingerers and subject to jail if unwilling to work. Before the Poor Laws, in the period following the enclosure of the common land and the resulting increase in unemployed persons travelling from town to town, distinctions needed to be made between those who were seen as entitled to beg—the worthy poor—and those not.[13] The former group, including "unmarried mothers, orphans, the mentally and physically disabled, and sick persons would live with kin or neighbors and be given food and fuel supplements from community resources. That a common social practice [of an earlier era] was formalized into the legal code [with the Poor Laws] is indicative of the broad social change caused by rapid urbanization" (Scheer & Groce, 1988, p. 32).

Despite an almost unending flow of laws following the codification of the Poor Laws in 1601, the problem of large numbers of unemployed persons moving around the country was not solved. Finally, in 1834, the Poor Law Amendment attempted to establish national standards; institute the principle that assistance would be denied to nondisabled persons outside of the workhouse (the prohibition on "outside" relief); and use deterrence as the basis for setting benefit levels (through the principle of "least eligibility," i.e., setting benefits levels below that of the lowest paid worker). The definition of those subject to the new Poor Law strictures was by elimination: those who were not children, sick people, persons with mental illness, "defectives," and the "aged and infirm." In effect, except

---

[13]While one society saw fit to make such distinctions, another did not. For example, among the Native American Creek, the original meaning of the word *haksi* is "'deaf' but it has come to signify 'drunken', 'roguish', 'wicked', 'sinful', etc." (Swanton, 1928, p. 339).

for the first group, these are people whom we now consider among persons with disabilities. "This strategy of definition by default remains at the core of current disability programs. None provides a positive definition of 'ablebodied;' instead, 'able to work' is a residual category whose meaning can be known only after all the 'unable to work' categories have been precisely defined" (Stone, 1984, pp. 40–41).

Over time, in the period following implementation of the Poor Laws, family and neighbors could no longer provide the resources necessary to sustain those within the category of the worthy poor; thus, the local government came to do so, usually contracting for provision of services with the lowest bidder in a public auction.

> The auction-contract system often resulted in neglect and abuse of the sick, disabled, and other persons in need of care. Beginning in the late 18th century, the American impotent poor were also sheltered in public almshouses. Although almshouses were planned to correct the abuses of the contract-auction system of care, institutional conditions were generally unsatisfactory. (Scheer & Groce, 1988, p. 33)

Rothman (1971) carefully tracks the change in care systems that came with the development of asylums. The nineteenth century development of the disease/medical model of care systems, replacing the earlier worthy poor concept, led first to asylums for persons with mental illness, and then to facilities for persons with blindness, with deafness, and with mental retardation.

> Although 19th-century asylums and 20th-century long-term rehabilitation hospitals reformed the type of institutional care available for disabled inmates of almshouses, the segregation, isolation, and infantilization of disabled patients continued. Since it had become customary to detach a portion of the disabled population from the mainstream of life, most Americans have lost familiarity with disabled people, so common in small-scale societies. (Scheer & Groce, 1988, p. 33)

Funk (1987), in a survey of the treatment of persons with disabilities in the United States, characterizes the period from the founding of the country until the second decade of the twentieth century as "From attic to warehouse." The middle decades of the twentieth century, he labels as a time of segregation and charitable care. He summarizes conditions by the end of the 1950s in the following list.

1. Existence of massive total-care institutions to house disabled persons deemed unable to function in organized society.
2. Board, care, training, and work institutions to house specific groups of disabled persons who were deemed trainable to educable, but also considered in need of segregated and structured surroundings because it was believed their handicap would not permit them to compete or function in society.
3. Provisions of public entitlements to persons with severe disabilities in order to provide an alternative to total-care institutions.
4. Provision of rehabilitation benefits to a larger and more varied population of disabled persons, including veterans, with the primary goal of assisting those who were deemed capable of obtaining gainful employment.
5. Massive increases in the number, size, and power of disability-specific research and charitable organizations.
6. Increase in the numbers and sophistication of a broad range of medical and rehabilitation professionals.
7. Increasing activity by disability-specific advocacy and education organizations involved in networking among their constituency and instrumental in developing state and federal legislation and policy to aid membership needs.
8. Early development of legislation and policy, primarily on the part of disability professionals, to expand the provision of rehabilitation services to disabled individuals for whom employment was not considered an obtainable objective.

The black civil rights efforts of the 1960s and 1970s had their effects upon the disability community—in the example of advocacy and protest they demonstrated, in the organizing model they presented, and in the development of approaches to legal and civil rights issues. These were decades of the passage of major legislation, particularly the Rehabilitation Act of 1973,[14] PL 93-112 (Scotch, 1984); the Education for All Handicapped Children Act, PL 94-142 (Lipsky & Gartner, 1989); and the expansion of both income-maintenance and rehabilitation

---

[14]Longmore (1987) offers a unique gloss to the meaning of the act's central provision, Section 504. "504 moved beyond . . . social welfare notions by viewing such devices and services [adaptive devices, such as wheelchairs and sign language interpreters] as simply different modes of functioning and departed from traditional civil rights concepts by defining them as legitimate permanent differential treatment necessary to achieve and maintain equal access. This perspective was the heart of the emerging disability rights ideology" (p. 363). For a similar view of differential treatment to achieve equality, see Funk (1987).

programs (Berkowitz, 1987). Equally important, they were decades of development of institutions within the disability community, many stemming from the efforts of the programs for college students with disabilities; particularly noteworthy was the establishment of the Center for Independent Living in Berkeley by students attending the University of California. Although ultimately not successful, the American Coalition of Citizens with Disabilities, founded in 1974, was the first crossdisability national advocacy organization.

CONCEPTUALIZATIONS OF THE PLACE IN SOCIETY OF PERSONS WITH DISABILITIES

Perhaps most consequential, in the last decade of the twentieth century, are changes in conceptualization of the meaning of disability. While differing handicapping conditions—sensory impairments, orthopedic impairments, neurological impairments, language and speech disabilities, and emotional disturbances—have particular consequences for the individuals involved, in each instance it is the interplay between the condition and the environment that determines the extent to which an impairment becomes a handicap. A building without ramps or elevators becomes closed to persons who use wheelchairs; the absence of ballots in Braille disenfranchises persons who are blind; the refusal of a school system to catheterize students with spina bifida excludes them from education with their peers. Of course, the installation of ramps does not restore to the person who had polio the use of his legs, nor does the presence of a Braille ballot give sight to the woman who is blind, nor does school-provided catheterization close the open spinal cord of the student with spina bifida. What these adjustments do is to mitigate the effect of the disability.

But even more than the physical environment, it is the attitudinal milieu that affects persons with disabilities. Attitudes are both immediate, as expressed in the treatment of persons with disabilities, and the bases for decisions about the environment—both physical and social. Thus, for example, it is the belief that students with handicapping conditions are incapable of learning or behaving appropriately that leads school systems to establish separate systems for them or to hold them to lesser standards than those for "normal" students

(Lipsky & Gartner, 1989). It is an all or nothing concept of disability that requires a person to "prove" total incapacity in order to gain entitlement to various benefit programs; it is a skewed sense of the "place" of persons with disabilities in the society that permits the maintenance of public and private facilities that in effect establish a system of separation; it is the inculcation in the belief systems of the persons with disabilities themselves that encourages attitudes of acquiescence, so that they seek sympathy and understanding rather than mobilizing for liberation and entitlement.

The sources of these concepts and the images they produce, for both persons with disabilities and those who do not have disabilities (persons whom the disability rights movement calls, "temporarily able-bodied"), are varied. They are in literature and art, on television and in the movies, in religious texts and school books. And from these sources, the artifacts of culture, they infect public attitudes and become reified in public policies (Gartner & Joe, 1987).

During the twentieth century, primarily in the Western world but increasingly in the Third World as well, the dominant view of disability has been rooted in a medical model. In Talcott Parsons' classic formulation (1951), the sick role has four main characteristics: 1) the patient is exempted from normal social obligations, 2) the patient is not held responsible for being sick, 3) the state of being sick is considered legitimate if 4) the patient cooperates with the legitimate sources of help and works toward recovery. When the sick person's condition is chronic, as in the case of disability, an otherwise fair exchange is transformed "into a restatement in scientific and apparently objective terms of the most oppressive traditional stereotypes about the social ability of handicapped people. . ." (Gliedman & Roth, 1980, p. 41). The sick person's grant of temporary exemption from normal role obligations becomes a permanent exclusion from normal opportunities. In addition, exclusion of patients from responsibility becomes a generalized unwillingness to take seriously the self-assertion of the person with a disability. This self-assertion is viewed as a symptom of maladjustment. [15] The sick role's insistence that the patient cooperate

---

[15]As we note in Chapter 3, the same thing is done to parents of children with disabilities; that is, they are "labeled" and marked as deficient, and when they protest, this is seen as an indication of their lack of appropriate adjustment, a phenomenon that Lipsky (1985) has identified as a "Catch 22."

with the helpgiver and work toward recovery becomes an acceptance of permanent tutelage of those whose ministration too often, in John McKnight's acute phrase, is in the form of "disabling help" (McKnight, 1977).

Longmore characterizes the "bargain" that society makes with persons with disabilities as follows: "The non-handicapped majority says in effect, 'we will extend to you provisional and partial toleration of your public presence—as long as you display a continuous cheerful striving toward normalization'" (cited in Johnson, 1989a, p. 6). "The Bargain gives disabled people something "useful" to do: get rehabilitated; strive to be normal" (Johnson, 1989a, p. 6).

As Hahn (1987, 1989) has pointed out, increasingly disability has come to be viewed from an economic vantage point. That is, the health-related impairment is seen as presenting a limitation on the amount of work a person can do, or conversely, as embodied in various social welfare programs, the extent to which an individual is entitled to support because she or he is incapable of working. "By focusing on the capacity to work almost at the expense of other life activities, this approach not only is unidimensional, but it also makes some unwarranted and untenable assumptions about the linkage between impairments and productivity" (Hahn, 1987, p. 182).

A later sociopolitical view of disability has been developed that considers disability a product of the interaction between the individual and the environment.

> Whereas both prior orientations regard disability as principally a personal misfortune, the sociopolitical approach stresses the role of the environment in determining the meaning of this phenomenon. . . . [A] comprehensive understanding of disability requires an examination of the architectural, institutional, and attitudinal environment encountered by persons with disabilities. From this perspective, the primary problems confronting citizens with disabilities are bias, prejudice, segregation, and discrimination that can be eradicated through policies designed to guarantee them equal rights. (Hahn, 1987, p. 182)

CONCEPTUALIZATIONS OF AESTHETICS AND OF ASPECTS OF WHAT IT MEANS TO BE HUMAN

Some within the disability rights movement have proposed a further view. Commenting on "The Bargain" described above,

Johnson (1989a), one of the founders of the movement's *Disability Rag*, says, "The Bargain . . . is a way of controlling a minority by forcing upon them the physical standards of the majority culture" (p. 8). Hahn (1988) has developed this notion most fully, arguing that prejudice and discrimination against persons with disabilities are rooted in an "aesthetic anxiety—the fear of others whose traits are perceived as disturbing or unpleasant" (p. 26). He argues, that "unlike other minorities, however, disabled men and women have not yet been able to refute implicit or direct accusations of biological inferiority" (p. 26) or, in Goffman's (1963) phrase, of being "not quite human" (p. 5).

> By reclaiming an aesthetic tradition that originated in one of the earliest eras of human history, and by overturning the moral order of the human body imposed by such authorities as the church and the mass media, it is possible to assert proudly that "disability is beautiful."
>
> Just as other disadvantaged groups have sometimes uncovered solutions to their problems by reexamining their own history, research on peoples with disabilities seemingly provides a solid foundation for the development of a positive sense of personal and political identity. For thousand of years, in a legacy that appeared to emerge from ancient fertility rites and that persisted until religious and economic interests managed to impose another order on the human body, the appearance of physical differences seemed to be associated with festiveness, sensuality, and entertainment rather than with loss, repugnance, or personal tragedy. These trends seem to form a sufficient basis for the redefinition of the identity of persons with disabilities. (Hahn, 1988, pp. 30–31)

Frank (1988) too, looks to the larger consequences of different understandings of disability. She notes that Fiedler (1978) "writes that truly physically variant human beings challenge the conventional boundaries between male and female, sexed and sexless, animal and human, large and small, and self and other" (p. 67). And reflecting on her study of a woman with a congenital limb impairment, she says:

> For me, the encounter with Diane challenged my adherence to the conventional linkages among physical normalcy, beauty, sexuality, and social integration. In addition, it evoked for me a heightened awareness of issues beyond elementary forms of social order, such as my own anxious feelings of helplessness and immobility, and lack and loss. The encounter with Diane further evoked an image of mythic beauty, the Venus de Milo, which, it

should be remembered, is the portrait of a goddess. (Frank, 1988, pp. 67–68)

And bringing us back full circle to the consideration of the effect of culture on the meaning of disability, Hahn (1988) points to the potential of accepting that "disability is beautiful" as enabling persons with disabilities to affect the society as a whole.

> Disabled people could play a significant role as critics of a culture that places inordinate stress on a rather conformist vision of external attractiveness and on a vain search for "the body beautiful." In a society that often seems to have gone berserk in a futile quest to achieve unattainable physical standards, women and men with disabilities may need to offer an alternative model of attraction that would permit both disabled and non-disabled persons to discover enhanced aesthetic satisfaction in the appearance of the ordinary men and women whom they encounter in everyday life. (p. 30)

Dennis Potter, the English television writer, who has severe attacks of psoriasis "that wrack his limbs and infest his skin, sending his body temperature soaring, sometimes to the point of inducing delirium" (Ward, 1988, p. 38), writes:

> It could be said that my illness, although my enemy, is also my ally, my ally in that it removes me from the hustle and bustle and makes me redefine myself.
> I've had to face questions that are embarrassing for a healthy man, especially a young man, about God and pain and humiliation. Those are questions normal people postpone asking. But when they come crashing in like the tide, there's no time not to answer them. Then maybe illness gives you something, too.[16] (Ward, 1988, p. 38)

Beyond the question of the intrinsic correctness or utility of particular ways of framing attention to issues of disability, Fine and Asch (1988), in their introduction to a special issue of the *Journal of Social Issues*, point out that reframing dis-

---

[16]An interesting parallel is found in the report about a soothsayer on Yap (an island in the Pacific), who fell from a coconut tree and injured his spine, and, as a result, spent over 2 years in his house with "no one to talk to; I think and I think over everything; I talk to myself; I remember the old stories" (Furness, 1910, p. 127). The visiting anthropologist notes, "This had been his school—two years of solitary self-conversation, and during this time he had pondered on the problems of nature and the human mind, and solved them in his simple primitive [sic] way, to his own satisfaction. He emerged a wise man, as they believed, with prophetic foresight" (p. 127).

ability as a minority group issue requires reanalysis in several dimensions:

1. How the experience of disability is influenced by professionals and how it can be studied by nondisabled researchers.
2. That disability needs to be studied over time and in context, as a socially transforming and changing process, not a static characteristic of an individual.
3. That a social-constructivist view of disability enables a reassessment of previously taken-for-granted views of the nature and consequences of life with impairment.
4. That accepting a minority-group perspective on disability and attending to all aspects of the life space that extend beyond the person with the impairment causes social psychologists to raise new questions for research. Examples of such questions include the following: What sustains the belief that having a child with a disability is predominantly burdensome and tragic? What would make possible a different outcome? What does the experience of being close to someone with a disability do to broaden one's sense of moral community or to shrink it? What are the consequences and costs, for both disabled and nondisabled people, of an increasingly integrated society? (p. 19)

CROSS-CULTURAL COMPARISONS

Few scholars have delved deeply enough into issues of culture and disability to provide cross-cultural analyses. Grand and Strohmer (1983) and Jordan (1971) report differences in attitudes toward disability among African-Americans as compared with white Americans, while Tseng (1972) contrasts the views of Asians to those of Americans. And several studies (Florian, 1982; Florian & Katz, 1983; Shurka & Florian, 1983) report significant differences between the attitudes toward disability among Israel's Jews and Arabs.

In examining the views toward disability of ethnic minorities in the United States, Florian (1987)[17] makes the point that it is important to understand the double minority status of these families when they have a member with a disability. He

---

[17]Florian brings to this analysis several valuable perspectives: that of an immigrant to his current homeland, Israel, where he has studied the differing responses to disabilities of Jews and Arabs; that of a frequent visitor to the United States, where he has studied the responses of ethnic minorities; and that of a person with a disability.

cites Chan's report (1976) that among Asian-Americans, particularly Chinese-Americans, the perception of persons with disabilities "as permanently unsound or incomplete individuals who have been cursed for sins committed by their ancestors" leads to "little interest in remedial therapy and places the onus on the family to care for less able members [sic]" (p. 43). And describing the people of Southeast Asia, Nguyen (1989) makes the same point:

> Traditionally, since people with disabilities are believed to be punishments to their families, the handicapped person is isolated from society, and is considered useless, worthless, a shame on the family. Nothing will be done for them. They have no future. (p. 11)

In discussing African-Americans, Florian (1987) cites studies that emphasize the importance of the family network responsible for all children (Ball, Warhiet, Vandiver, & Holzer, 1979; Stack, 1974; Turnbull, Summers, & Brotherson, 1984), as well as a study (Wallace, 1980, cited in Florian, 1987) that reports African-American mothers' "positive attitudes toward the maintenance of their retarded children at home and satisfaction toward the reactions of family, friends, and community" (p. 43). In discussing Mexican-American families, he notes that they too have strong family ties, along with a relaxed attitude toward developmental milestones that encourages lengthy dependence upon the family (Falicov, 1982). Religious beliefs often lead to a fatalistic acceptance of the child with a disability (Marion, 1980) and sometimes a tendency to delay referral for appropriate intervention (Kunce, 1983). Rodriguez (1989) emphasizes the sense of isolation produced by the birth of a child with a disability, and "the deep fear and shame of subnormality" (p. 13).

In describing the situation in Israel, Florian (1987) contrasts not only the views of Arabs and Jews, but among Jews, differences between those of Western and Oriental origin, the latter's views being closer to those of the Arabs. Jews of Oriental origin appear to have more negative attitudes toward disability than do those of Western origin, and Arabs appear to have less positive attitudes than do either group of Jews. Florian examines these differences through the lenses of "shame" versus "guilt."

> The Israeli Jewish societal reaction to physical disability, characterized by a sense of guilt and consequently a strong sense of

responsibility, limits the impact of the spread effect. According to Wright (1982) this spread effect is often the core of negative attitudes toward the disabled. Thus the sense of guilt may, in fact, generate more positive attitudes. In contrast, what pressures the Arab is probably not guilt but shame, or more precisely the psychological drive to escape or prevent negative judgment by others. It may be suggested that this sensitivity to what others have to say predisposes more negative attitudes toward a person who displays deviant behaviour and/or deviant body characteristics. (p. 45)

And in comparing the response of parents of Jewish children with disabilities, "those of Western origin tended to blame medical negligence for the child's condition, whereas the parents of Oriental origin tended to blame fate or themselves" (p. 45).

CONCLUSION

While the importance of culture in understanding human behavior generally is recognized, often it is seen as a peripheral factor, not as significant as more "scientific" factors. Yet White (1988) points out:

It is still the case that only about 15 percent of all contemporary clinical interventions are supported by objective scientific evidence that they do more good than harm. On the other hand, between 40 and 60 percent of all therapeutic benefits can be attributed to a combination of the placebo and Hawthorne effects, two code words for caring and concern. . . . (pp. 9–10)

He goes on to point out that the book for which he is writing a Foreword (Payer, 1988) "provides chapter and verse at both the macro and micro levels to make the case that differences in national character and professional responses to patients' problems are important determinants of clinical care" (p. 10). He emphasizes the importance of "values [and] underlying paradigms" (p. 10). Illustrative of their importance are the data reported by Pliskin (1987) about the response of Israeli doctors to Iranian patients. Her argument centers on the traditional concept of "narahati," a term used by Iranians to connote undifferentiated, unpleasant, emotional and physical feelings. Although emotional manifestations of narahati are disapproved of, its expression as physical illness is not; thus, feelings of stress, for example, are often somatized. In noting aspects of the patients' situation and how it is addressed, Pliskin links this cultural origin of the Iranian patients' problems to the Israeli doctors' stereotypes about Iranians, which portray them as stupid, lazy, suspicious, stingy, primitive, and deceptive. The doctors apply these stereotypes when faced with diffuse physical symptoms that they cannot diagnose, thus creating a way to cope with the discomfort and anger they feel in their powerlessness to make use of their usual professional skill.

Just as the issues facing Israeli doctors in treating Iranian immigrants illustrate the relation between cultural perceptions and medical care, an examination of psychological treatment of new immigrants to the United States finds culture key in therapy (Goleman, 1989). The author cites a Harvard Medical School professor, Arthur Kleinman, who says, "The ethnocentric arrogance of Western psychotherapy is being challenged head on by the growing recognition of the problems in treating non-Western immigrants." Also, a New York City psychoanalyst, Alan Roland, writes, "The prevailing psychological maps we assume in the West to be universal simply do not apply to people in much of the world" (Goleman, 1989, pp. C1–6). Thus, some emotional problems occur in parts of the world but not in others. For example, agoraphobia and anorexia occur only in Western countries.

Reactions to two tragedies in the United States make explicit the point about the pertinence of culture. In January, 1989, in Stockton, California, a gunman killed five children in a school playground, all of them Southeast Asian refugees. In commenting upon the problems of helping the community to heal, considering both Southeast Asian and white Americans, a school psychologist says, "What one culture considers help, the other culture considers an imposition—or just plain bizarre" (Gross, 1989, p. A18). Thus, "while white families have clamored for more help for themselves and their children, the Asians are bewildered by the parade of social workers and psychiatrists asking them how they feel" (p. A18). "'We would rather go to a friend, a relative, a monk,' said Sophan Thong, a counselor at the Cambodian Community, a refugee center. . . . 'You keep each other company, talk about this, talk about that and forget your tragedy'" (p. A18). The school's principal has made great efforts to understand the Asian community's needs, including those that grew out of their Buddhist beliefs that the playground remains inhabited by the ghosts of those killed; she arranged a ceremony to rid the playground of ghosts. This has led some of the white families to criticize her for bending over backwards for the Southeast Asians.

In New York City, a recent Chinese immigrant, who killed his wife, was given a lenient sentence (5 years of probation) by a judge, who relied upon the testimony of a college professor who testified that Chinese marriages are considered so sacred that husbands in China often exact severe punishment on wives who admit to adultery. When the prosecutor decried the judge's leniency, some Asian-American groups "expressed outrage because they said it cast a shadow on Chinese culture. 'We have always wanted a more culturally informed judicial system, but this case completely crosses the line—to the point of excusing a murder,'" said Monona Yin, from the Committee Against Anti-Asian violence" (Bohlen, 1989, p. B4). A Brooklyn Law School professor (Herman, 1989) argues that while culture should not be an absolute defense, it should be a factor in considering the cause of the behavior and, on occasion, as in this case, mitigating the punishment. She buttresses her argument by noting that the criminal justice system has accepted other defenses, including insanity, post-traumatic stress syndrome, menstrual stress, and so forth, and, therefore, accepting "culture not as a complete defense but as a factor in sentencing is a reasonable one" (p. B4).

The point concerning families and supports for families with a child who has disabilities is that to provide supports appropriately requires cultural understanding of both the meaning of disability and the nature and roles of families and ways in which they can be supported. It is to this latter set of issues that we turn in Chapter 3.

REFERENCES

Agosta, J., O'Neal, M., & Toubbeh, J. (Eds.). (1987). *A path to peace of mind: Providing exemplary services to Navajo children with developmental disabilities and their families.* Window Rock, AZ: Save the Children Federation, Navajo Nation Field Office.

Asch, A. (1988a). Disability: Its place in the psychology curriculum. In P.A. Bronstein & K. Quina (Eds.), *Teaching a psychology of people: Resources for gender and sociocultural awareness* (pp. 156–167). Washington, DC: American Psychological Association.

Asch, A. (1988b). Reproductive technology and disability. In S. Cohen & N. Taub (Eds.), *Reproductive laws for the 1990's*. Clifton, NJ: Humana Press.

Ball, R., Warhiet, G., Vandiver, J., & Holzer, C. (1979). Kin ties of low-income Blacks and Whites. *Ethnicity, 6*, 184–196.

Belenky, M.B., Clinchy, B.M., Goldberger, N.R., & Tarule, J.M. (1986). *Women's ways of knowing: The development of self, voice, and mind*. New York: Basic Books.

Berkowitz, E.D. (1987). *Disabled policy: America's programs for the handicapped*. A Twentieth Century Fund Report. Cambridge: Cambridge University Press.

Biklen, D. (1989). Making difference ordinary. In S. Stainback, W. Stainback, & M. Forest (Eds.), *Educating all students in the mainstream of regular education* (pp. 235–248). Baltimore: Paul H. Brookes Publishing Co.

Biklen, D. (n.d.). *The culture of policy: Disability images in literature and their analogue in public policy*. Unpublished manuscript, Syracuse University, Syracuse, New York.

Birdsell, J.D. (1972). *Human evolution: An introduction to the new physical anthropology*. Chicago: Rand McNally.

Bogdan, R. (1980). What does it mean when a person says, 'I am not retarded'? *Education and Training of the Mentally Retarded 15*, 74–79.

Bohlen, C. (1989, April 5). Light sentence in husband's slaying of wife stirs outrage. *New York Times*, p. B4.

Browne, S., Connors, D., & Stern, N. (1985). *With the power of each breath: A disabled women's anthology*. Pittsburgh: Cleis Press.

Brozan, N. (1988, August 7). Gay groups are rallied to aid 2 women's fight. *New York Times*, p. 26.

Bulwer, J. (1648). *Philocophus: Or the deafe and dumbe mans friend*. London: Humphrey Moseley.

Burnet, J. R. (1835). *Tales of the deaf and dumb*. Newark: Benjamin Olds.

Carver V., & Rodda, M. (1978). *Disability and the environment*. New York: Schocken Books.

Chan, D.C. (1976). Asian-American handicapped people: An area of concern. *Journal of Rehabilitation, 42*(6), 14–16.

Cole, M., Gay, J., Glick, J.A., & Sharp, D.W. (1971). *The cultural context of learning and thinking: An exploration in experimental anthropology*. New York: Basic Books.

Deegan, M.J., & Brooks, N.A. (1985). *Women and disability: The double handicap*. New Brunswick, NJ: Transaction Books.

Driedger, D. (1989). *The last civil rights movement: Disabled Peoples' International*. New York: St. Martin's Press.

Dybwad, G. (1970). Treatment of the mentally retarded: A cross-national view. In H.C. Haywood (Ed.), *Social-cultural aspects of mental retardation* (pp. 560–572). New York: Appleton-Century-Crofts.

Eckholm, E. (1989, January 8). River blindness: Conquering an ancient scourge. *New York Times*, pp. 20–27, 58–61.

Edgerton, R.B. (1970). Mental retardation in non-Western societies: Toward a cross-cultural perspective on incompetence. In H.C. Haywood (Ed.), *Social-cultural aspects of mental retardation* (pp. 523–559). New York: Appleton-Century-Crofts.

Edgerton, R.B., & Langness, L.L. (1974). *Methods and styles in the study of culture.* San Francisco: Chandler & Sharp Publishers.

Falicov, C.J. (1982). Mexican families. In M. McGoldrick, J.K. Pearce, & J. Giordano (Eds.), *Ethnicity in family therapy.* New York: The Guilford Press.

Fiedler, L. (1978). *Freaks.* New York: Simon & Schuster.

Fine, M., & Asch, A. (1985). Disabled women: Sexism without the pedestal. In M.J. Deegan & N.A. Brooks (Eds.), *Women and disability: The double handicap.* New Brunswick, NJ: Transaction Books.

Fine, M., & Asch, A. (1988). Disability beyond stigma: Social interaction, discrimination, and activism. *Journal of Social Issues, 44*(1), 3–21.

Fine, M., & Asch, A. (1989). *Women with disabilities: Essays in psychology, culture, and politics.* Philadelphia: Temple University Press.

Florian, V. (1982). Cross-cultural differences in attitudes toward disabled persons—A study of Jewish and Arab youth in Israel. *International Journal of Intercultural Relations, 6,* 291–299.

Florian, V. (1987). Family supports in Israel. In D.K. Lipsky (Ed.), *Family supports for families with a disabled member* (pp. 37–55) (Monograph No. 39). New York: World Rehabilitation Fund.

Florian, V., & Katz, S. (1983). The impact of cultural, ethnic, and national variables on attitudes toward the disabled in Israel: A review. *International Journal of Intercultural Relations, 7,* 167–179.

Frank, G. (1988). On embodiment: A case study of congenital limb deficiency in American culture. In M. Fine & A. Asch (Eds.), *Women with disabilities: Essays in psychology, culture, and politics* (pp. 41–71). Philadelphia: Temple University Press.

Freud, S. (1920). *The interpretation of dreams.*

Funk, R., (1987). Disability rights: From case to class in the context of civil rights. In A. Gartner & T. Joe (Eds.), *Images of the disabled/disabling images* (pp. 7–30). New York: Praeger.

Furness, W.H. (1910). *The island of stone money: Uap of the Carolines.* Philadelphia: J.B. Lippincott.

Gallagher, H.G. (1985). *FDR's splendid deception.* New York: Dodd, Mead.

Gardner, H. (1983). *Frames of mind: The theory of multiple intelligences.* New York: Basic Books.

Gartner, A., & Joe, T. (1987). *Images of the disabled/disabling images.* New York: Praeger.

Gartner, A., & Lipsky, D.K. (1989). Beyond special education: Toward a quality system for all students. *Harvard Educational Review, 57*(4), 367–395.

Giami, A. (1987). Coping with sexuality of the disabled: A comparison of the physically disabled and the mentally retarded. *International Journal of Rehabilitation Research, 10*(1), 41–48.

Gilligan, C. (1979). Women's place in man's life cycle. *Harvard Educational Review, 49,* 431–436.

Gliedman, J., & Roth, W. (1980). *The unexpected minority: Handicapped children in America.* New York: Harcourt, Brace, Jovanovich.

Goffman, E. (1963). *Stigma: Notes on the management of spoiled identity.* Englewood Cliffs, NJ: Prentice-Hall.

Goldman, J., & Gardner, H. (1989). Multiple paths to educational effectiveness. In D.K. Lipsky & A. Gartner (Eds.), *Beyond separate education: Quality education for all* (pp. 121–139). Baltimore: Paul H. Brookes Publishing Co.

Goleman, D. (1989, March 7). The self: From Tokyo to Topeka, it changes. *New York Times,* p. C1.

Grand, S.A., & Strohmer, D.C. (1983). Minority perceptions of the disabled. *Rehabilitation Bulletin,* 117–119.

Groce, N.E. (1985). *Everyone here spoke sign language: Hereditary deafness on Martha's Vineyard.* Cambridge, MA: Harvard University Press.

Gross, J. (1989, May 21). Survivors heal slowly where 5 children died. *New York Times,* p. A18.

Gwaltney, J.L. (1970). *The thrice shy: Cultural accommodation to blindness and other disasters in a Mexican community.* New York: Columbia University Press.

Hahn, H. (1987). Civil rights for disabled Americans: The foundation of a political agenda. In A. Gartner & T. Joe (Eds.), *Images of the disabled/disabling images* (pp. 181–204). New York: Praeger.

Hahn, H. (1988). Can disability be beautiful? *Social Policy, 19* (3), 26–32.

Hahn, H. (1989). The politics of special education. In D.K. Lipsky & A. Gartner (Eds.). *Beyond separate education: Quality education for all* (pp. 225–241). Baltimore: Paul H. Brookes Publishing Co.

Hanks, J.R., & Hanks, L.M. (1948). The physically handicapped in certain non-Occidental societies. *Journal of Social Issues 4,* 11–20.

Herman, S.N. (1989, April 20). Should culture be a defense? *Newsday,* p. 80.

Jenkins, W.G. (1890). The scientific testimony of 'facts and opinions'. *American Annals of the Deaf, 35*(3), 184–191.

Jernigan, K. (1985, August-September). Presidential address. *Braille Monitor,* p. 387.

Johnson, M. (1989a). The bargain. *Disability Rag, 10*(5), 5–6.

Johnson, M. (1989b). Tin cups and Tiny Tim. *Disability Rag, 10*(5), 9–10.

Jordan, J.E. (1971). Attitude-behavior research on physical-mental-social disability and racial-ethnic differences. *Psychological Aspects of Disability 18*(1), 5–26.

Jung, C.G. (1916). *Psychology of the unconscious.* London: Keegan Paul.

Karuth, D. (1985). If I were a car, I'd be a lemon. In A. Brightman (Ed.), *Ordinary moments: The disabled experience* (pp. 9–31). Syracuse, NY: Human Policy Press.

Kent, D. (1987). Disabled women: Portraits in fiction and drama. In A. Gartner & T. Joe (Eds.), *Images of the disabled/disabling images* (pp. 47–64). New York: Praeger.

Kent, D. (1989). In search of a heroine: Images of women with disabilities in fiction and drama. In M. Fine & A. Asch (Eds.), *Women with disabilities: Essays in psychology, culture, and politics* (pp. 90–110). Philadelphia: Temple University Press.

Kriegel, L. (1987). The cripple in literature. In A. Gartner & T. Joe (Eds.), *Images of the disabled/ disabling images* (pp. 31–46). New York: Praeger.

Kristof, N.D. (1989, July 19). Change comes to North Korea, ever so reluctantly. *New York Times,* pp. A2.

Kuhn, T. K. (Ed.). (1962). *The structure of scientific revolutions.* Chicago: University of Chicago Press.

Kunce, J.T. (1983). *The Mexican-Americans: Cross-cultural rehabilitation counseling implications.* Final report for the World Rehabilitation Fund. New York: The Fund.

Lane, H. (1984). *When the mind hears: A history of the deaf.* New York: Random House.

Lane, H. (1988). Is there a "psychology of the deaf"? *Exceptional Children, 55*(1), 7–19.

Langness, L. L. (1987). *The study of culture.* Novato, CA: Chandler & Sharp Publishers.

Liachowitz, C.H. *Disability as a social construct.* Philadelphia: University of Pennsylvania Press.

Lipsky, D.K. (1985). A parental perspective on stress and coping. *American Journal of Orthopsychiatry, 55*(4), 614–617.

Lipsky, D.K., & Gartner, A. (Eds.). (1989). *Beyond separate education: Quality education for all.* Baltimore: Paul H. Brookes Publishing Co.

Longmore, P.K. (1987). Uncovering the hidden histories of people with disabilities. *Reviews in American History,* 355–364.

Mann, E.J. (1836). *The deaf and dumb or, A collection of articles relating to the condition of deaf-mutes, their education and the principal asylums devoted to their instruction.* Boston: D.K. Hithcock.

Marion, R.L. (1980). Communicating with parents of culturally diverse exceptional children. *Exceptional Children, 46,* 616–623.

McKnight, J. (1977). Professional service and disabling help. In A. Brechin, P. Liddiard, & J. Swain (Eds.), *Handicap in social world.* London: Open University Press.

Mead, M. (1928). *Coming of age in Samoa.* New York: William Morrow.

Mercer, J.R. (1988). Death of the IQ paradigm: Where do we go from here? In W.L. Lonner & V.O. Tyler (Eds.), *Cultural and ethnic factors in learning and motivation: Implications for education* (pp. 1–21). Pullman, WA: Western Washington University.

Miles, M. (1983). Why Asia rejects Western disability advice. *Quad Wrangle, 6.*

Miller, G.A. (1971). Foreword. In M. Cole, J. Gay, J.A. Glick, & D.W. Sharp. *The cultural context of learning and thinking.* New York: Basic Books.

Murdock, G.P. (1949). *Social structure.* New York: The Free Press.

Murdock, G.P. (1965). *Culture and society.* Pittsburgh: University of Pittsburgh Press.

Nguyen, D.Q. (1989). An overview of Southeast Asian culture. *Coalition Quarterly, 6*(2, 3), 10–11.

Nolan, C. (1987). *Under the eye of the clock.* New York: Delta.

Parsons, T. (1951). *The social system.* Glencoe, IL: Free Press.

Payer, L. (1988). *Medicine & culture: Varieties of treatment in the United States, England, West Germany, and France.* New York: Henry Holt.

Pliskin, K.L. (1987). *Silent boundaries: Cultural constraints on sickness and diagnosis of Iranians in Israel.* New Haven: Yale University Press.

Rapp, R. (1988). Moral pioneers: Women, men, and fetuses on a frontier of reproductive technology. In E.H. Baruch, A. D'Adamo, & J. Seager (Eds.), *Embryos, ethics and women's rights: Exploring the new reproductive technologies* (pp. 101–116). New York: The Haworth Press.

Rodriguez, J.R. (1989). Hispanic culture. *Coalition Quarterly, 6* (2, 3), 12–14.

Rothman, D. (1971). *The discovery of the asylum: Social order and disorder in the New Republic.* Boston: Little, Brown.

Rowe, J.H. (1946). Inca culture at the time of the Spanish conquest. *Bureau of American Ethnology Bulletin, 142*(2), 183–330.

Saxton, M. (1985). The something that happened before I was born. In A. Brightman (Ed.), *Ordinary moments: The disabled experience* (pp. 127–140). Syracuse: Human Policy Press.

Scheer, J., & Groce, N. (1988). Impairment as a human constant: Cross-cultural and historical perspectives on variation. *Journal of Social Issues, 44*(1), 23–37.

Scotch, R.K. (1984). *From good will to civil rights: Transforming federal disability policy.* Philadelphia: Temple University Press.

Seiss, J.A. (1887). *The children of silence or, the story of the deaf.* Philadelphia: Porter and Coates.

Shurka, E., & Florian, V. (1983). A study of Israeli Jewish and Arab perceptions of their child with a disability. *Journal of Comparative Family Studies, 14*(3), 367–375.

Solomon, W.S. (1987, November 29). Deaf writer asks questions that echo for young. *New York Times,* p. 68.

Sontag, S. (1979). *Illness as metaphor.* New York: Random House.

Stack, C. (1974). *All our kin: Strategies for surviving in a black community.* New York: Harper & Row.

Stone, D.A. (1984). *The disabled state.* Philadelphia: Temple University Press.

Swanton, J.R. (1928). *Social organization and social usages of the Indians of the Creek Confederacy.* Forty-second Annual Report of the Bureau of American Ethnology. Washington, DC: Government Printing Office.

Tobin, J.T., Wu, D.Y.H., & Davidson, D.H. (1989). Preschool education in three cultures. *Education Week, 9*(3), 26.

Tseng, M.S. (1972). Attitudes toward the disabled: A cross-cultural study. *The Journal of Social Psychology, 87,* 311–326.

Turnbull, A.P., Summers, J.A., & Brotherson, M.J. (1984). *Working with families with a member with a disability: A family systems approach.* Lawrence, KS: University Affiliated Facility.

Wallace, B. J. (1980). *Black mothers' attitudes toward their disabled children.* Doctoral dissertation, Brandeis University.

Ward, A. (1988, November 13). TV's tormented master. *New York Times,* p. 38.

White, K.L. (1988). Foreword. In L. Payer (Ed.). *Medicine and culture: Varieties of treatment in the United States, England, West Germany, and France.* New York: Henry Holt.

Wright, B.A. (1982). *Physical disability: A psychosocial approach* (2nd ed.). New York: Harper & Row.

Zola, I.K. (1985). Depictions of disability—Metaphor, message, and medium in the media: A research and political agenda. *The Social Science Journal, 22*(4), 5–17.

3

Families and a Child with a Disability

The most important thing that happens when a child is born with disabilities is that a child is born. The most important thing that happens when a couple becomes parents of a child with disabilities is that a couple becomes parents. (Ferguson & Asch, 1989, p. 108)

To recognize that families are important in the life of a child with disabilities, and vice versa, is to say no more—and no less—than what is true of all families and all children. And yet, somehow this is seen as a unique understanding. In part, this is because, as with children with disabilities, the family is labeled as special, with the connotation of defective, indeed disabled (Lipsky, 1985). Also, this understanding grows out of the proclivity, at least in societies with developed social welfare systems (and those that wish to emulate them), to respond to needs with formal services, the antonym of natural settings of family and community. Furthermore, what otherwise might be seen as "normal" developments, for example, tension at transition points, becomes pathologized and thus, requires formal services.

This is not to say that families with a child with a disability do not have needs; they may. But in understanding and addressing those needs, it is appropriate, we believe, to recognize that first, these families are more alike than different from other families, and second, that every family at differing times has particular needs (Lipsky, 1989), perhaps even at the birth of the first child, whether the child does or does not have disabilities. Indeed, research suggests that 50% of couples report less marital satisfaction after the birth of their first child (Rubenstein, 1989).

And, just as it is necessary to recognize that each family is different and individual, so too, it is necessary to recognize that the perspectives and interests of family members are different and individual.

> The perspective of parents is notoriously different from that of their children regardless of whether the children are disabled or not. Not surprisingly, then, the narratives of parents of disabled children sometimes emphasize different aspects of events than do accounts of disabled adults recalling their childhood. (Ferguson & Asch, 1989, p. 111)

This point is illustrated uniquely in *Retarded ISN'T Stupid, Mom!* (Kaufman, 1988), which combines the perspectives of the author, in her roles as both ethnographer and mother, and her daughter, who has mild mental retardation.

Not only are there differences in the perspectives of children and parents, the data available about the experiences of children with disabilities and of families with a child with disabilities also vary.

> The list of disabilities represented in the parent narratives is different from that represented in the individual autobiographies [of persons with disabilities]. Most mentally retarded children, for example, do not write books or articles when they grow up. Many parents, however, have written about mental retardation. On the other hand, comparatively few parent narratives exist describing life with a child who is blind, although there is a significant group of narratives written by blind adults. (Ferguson & Asch, 1989, p. 111)

LABELING PARENTS

The observation that handicapped children generally make handicapped parents is almost a cliche today. (McDonald, 1979, p. 44)

If the families of handicapped children can be salvaged, the children can probably be salvaged, too. (Reid, 1979, p. 61)

As children with disabilities are labeled, so too, are their parents. Just as the patient with a disease of the liver becomes, in the flip phrase of the hospital personnel, "the liver," the parents of a child with spina bifida become the "spina bifida parents." "Thus, parents often become a curious trait usually associated with the disability under investigation, whether mental retardation, blindness, autism, or perhaps just handicaps in general" (Ferguson & Asch, 1989, p. 108). The damaging consequences of labeling for the child are extended to the parents as well (Ferguson & Ferguson, 1987; Sarason & Doris, 1979).

The problem is not only that parents are labeled; the same model of pathology that is used in describing the child with a disability is applied to the parents as well. Just as the handicaps the child faces are ascribed solely to the impairment, not to the societal response, the parents' reactions are also seen in an intrapsychic mode, a melange of shock, sorrow, denial, and rejection. The parents' reactions are never viewed as rational responses to the burdens imposed by inadequate services, the insults of professional ignorance, or the lack of social and economic supports (Lipsky, 1985). Indeed, it is rare to find in the professional literature reports of parents' positive adaptive responses. It is rare to find reports reflecting, as we discuss below, the recognition that variations in family responses are more a function of factors such as culture or economic situation, than they are a function of whether or not there is a child with a disability in the family.

As Gliedman and Roth (1980) have pointed out, professionals have evolved a social pathology paradigm to describe and explain parental behavior. It includes the following aspects:

> Overprotection and idealization are used by parents to avoid the reality of the disability.
> Insistence on obtaining full information and services is "shopping around" for an alternative diagnosis in order to deny the reality of the handicap.
> Parental depression is the result of incomplete grief over the loss of the idealized child.
> Guilt, rage, and hostility are frequent dynamics in the family with a disabled member.

> Parents who cope successfully and remain optimistic are over-compensating to diminish their sense of guilt.
> Family dysfunction results from inadequate emotional adjust-ment to bearing an "eternal child." (MacKinnon & Marlett, 1984, p. 113)

Lusthaus (n.d.) has catalogued the professional literature's ascription of parental responses and offered interesting alter-native explanations. To the shock that is most often described, she counterposes the point that: "In refusing to consider disap-pointment and tragedy as normal modes of existence . . . we magnify frustration and suffering for families with a disabled child" (p. 36). Accepting these normal modes of existence does not require a disregard of reality. As one parent (Pieper, n.d.) writes:

> Jeff is neither my burden nor my chastisement, although his care requires more than I want to give at times. He is not an angel sent for my personal growth or my future glory; he is not a punishment for my past sins. He is a son. (p. 88)

The parent narratives of the 1940s and 1950s, and some later ones, often express a sense of spiritual growth as a result of having a child with disabilities. Some of this is reflected in the reports of the newly established Beach Center on Families and Disability at the University of Kansas in Lawrence. In an analysis of the letters sent by persons with disabilities or by their family members to the United States Department of Health and Human Services as comments upon the 1983 pro-posed regulations concerning the medical treatment of new-borns with disabilities (the "Baby Jane Doe Regulations"), the University of Kansas researchers found that

> virtually all of these letter writers supported the regulations and some 35 percent supported their points by describing at least one positive contribution the person with a disability had made to others, including being a source of: joy to the family, learning life's lessons, love, blessing or fulfillment, pride, strengthening the family. (Disability and the family, 1989, p. 1. For a fuller discus-sion of this topic, cf. Turnbull, Guess, & Turnbull, 1988.)

Later narratives, and some earlier ones, "describe a family life of increased tolerance of differences, and a heightened awareness of the daily injustices needlessly dealt out by our society to people in one minority group or another" (Ferguson & Asch, 1989, p. 113).

Speaking of his son, who has severe mental retardation, Ferguson says,

> As a father, I do not love my son *in spite* [italics in the original] of his handicaps as some abstracted, idealized version of reality. The object of my affection is the flesh and blood Ian whom I dress every day, put in a wheelchair, and struggle to talk to in words he can understand. (Ferguson & Asch, 1989, p. 114)

Most parents of children with disabilities have acknowledged feeling sorrow in varying degrees at various times. While there is little research to substantiate their feelings of happiness,[1] many parents express a mixture of joy as well as sorrow. And at particular developmental benchmarks or transition points, there may be a heightened sense of one or the other emotion. When parents do not express sorrow, or express too much joy, however, they are often viewed as being in denial.

Denial is a complex phenomenon that ranges from denying existence of the handicap altogether to minimizing its severity to over-involvement in dealing with the disability. Of course, as Lusthaus (n.d.) points out: "parents can be mistakenly accused of denial when they have a legitimate difference with professional opinion" (p. 9). And the often criticized "shopping around" behavior may in other contexts be seen as an appropriate form of seeking a second (or third) opinion.

A different perspective on parents visiting many different doctors is expressed in a publication of The National Society for Children and Adults with Autism (1981):

> The pediatric clinic says that the child is "slow in developing," the parents must wait. Try a mental retardation specialist.
> The mental retardation specialist finds the child is not testable. It must be a brain dysfunction. Try pediatric neurology.
> Pediatric neurology comes up with "funny squiggles" on the EEG. Nothing specific. See a psychiatrist.
> The psychiatrist decides the child is too ill for testing and must be retarded. Try special education.
> Special education refers the child back to the pediatric clinic for diagnosis and treatment. (pp. 18f.)

The other side of denial is over-involvement or inappropriate involvement. The child, or her or his disability, becomes a

---

[1]Two collections, Simons (1987) and Turnbull and Turnbull (1978), offer reflections by parents of children with a range of disabilities.

"project." As Asch (Ferguson & Asch, 1989) points out: "making the child's disabilities and differences into a project [loses] sight of the rest of the child . . ." (p. 118). Speaking about herself and her parents, she says, "[Disability] was something that had to be thought about and contended with, sometimes it got them and me into humorous situations, and at other times it provoked struggle, but it never was what our relationship was about" (p. 120).

As Gallagher indicates (1956), parents are put into an untenable position when discussing rejection. If they express the honest feelings of not liking their child—as if only parents of a child with a disability ever have such feelings[2]—they are condemned for rejecting their child. If they say they like and love their child, they are viewed as unrealistic. The constant analyzing of parental behavior by professionals often produces parental anger. And, then, this too is analyzed.

> The belief that parents displace their anger onto the professional is a kind of "Catch 22." That is, whenever the parent disagrees with or confronts the professional, that behavior can be dismissed as an expression of inadequate adjustment, frustration, displaced anger, or a host of psychological problems. Any interpretation is possible other than the parent may be correct. (Lipsky, 1985, p. 616)

In discussing the literature concerning family adaptation to a child with a disability, Sabbeth and Leventhal (1984) note that of the studies they examined in an extensive review, more than two-thirds did not include a control group of families with a child who did not have a disability. In a carefully designed study with such a control group, Florian (1989) reports that, while there were some differences between families with and those without a child with a disability, the more central finding was that "The impact of having a child with a disability among Israeli Jewish families did not appear to have a differential influence on the dynamic patterns between parents with and without such a child" (p. 108). He views his finding as confirm-

---

[2]Wright (1983) elaborates on this point, writing that "parents love and hate . . . [handicapped] children just as parents love and hate children who are not physically impaired. Parents protect, guide wisely, pamper, neglect, and even abandon children whether or not they are handicapped. Some children were unwanted, but are loved and have the security of a healthy relationship with their parents. Some children were wanted, but are unloved and insecure, whether or not they are sound of mind and body" (p. 291).

ing the conclusion of Vance, Fazan, Satterwhite, and Pless (1980) that: "The more care an investigator takes in providing a control group and matching the samples, the less likely the results will demonstrate marked differences in functioning between families with handicapped children and healthy [sic] children" (p. 61). A similar conclusion is reached by Gallagher, Scharfman, and Bristol (1984) based upon a study comparing parents of preschool children with moderate to severe handicaps with parents of nonhandicapped preschool children. "A somewhat surprising result of this comparison was the very close relationships between the division of responsibilities in the families with the nonhandicapped and handicapped children" (Gallagher & Bristol, 1989, p. 297).

PARENT RESPONSE TO ATTITUDES AND SERVICES—IN THE UNITED STATES

MacKinnon and Marlett (1984) note changes in services in the United States across decades. In the middle of the nineteenth century, when persons with disabilities were first recognized as a distinct group, attitudes were similar to current thinking in the rehabilitation field: persons with disabilities were to be given the opportunity to develop to their full potential in a controlled world (Kanner, 1964). By the end of the century, however, the public attitude became more one of pity and charity and a protective institutional model was developed. With the growth of the eugenics movement, the institutional approach gained dominance (Rothman, 1971).

In the 1950s, parents of children with mental retardation began to rebel against forced institutionalization of their children. Against the advice of professionals, some parents kept their children at home and fought to establish services in the community. Parents came to see professionals as among their greatest problems (Darling, 1979) because they withheld information or delivered it in an insensitive manner,[3] and seemed to blame parents for their child's condition, especially if the parents refused to institutionalize the child. While we have talked

---

[3]Speaking at a New York City conference of The Association for Persons with Severe Handicaps (TASH), the father of a boy with disabilities said: "You don't need a doctor who will tell you what you want to hear. You need a doctor who will listen to what you say" (Kellerman, 1989).

about parents, in fact, it was mothers who provided most of the care and who were saddled with most of the blame (cf. Ehlers, 1966).

By the 1960s, parent-sponsored community services were being developed as an alternative to institutionalization. Although negative experiences with professionals continued, some parents, particularly those with children with physical disabilities, were receiving more help from the medical community. However, in many instances the professionals involved in these parent-organized programs "essentially ignored and devalued the family as a focal point of helping children with severe handicaps" (Lehr, 1987, p. 3). Although as yet still faint, the echoes of the black civil rights movement began to affect the consciousness of some persons with disabilities, and brought about the emergence of challenges to the conceptualization of disability as an illness that required abrogation of control that people were allowed over their own lives.

In the 1970s, a series of legislative mandates established the rights of persons with disabilities. Particularly in education, this legislation was the work of parents, along with persons with disabilities themselves and a small cadre of professionals. As these laws took effect, parents seemed to feel "less need to band together to fight the system. [S]ome parents' organizations report a 'generation gap'; younger parents do not identify with the crusading stance taken by older parents and often withdraw from organizations" (MacKinnon & Marlett, 1984, p. 118).

In the 1980s, three streams of development have moved forward: 1) an increasingly enlarged professional sphere, 2) an emergent movement among persons with disabilities themselves, although in many ways still quiescent, and 3) a continuing parents' struggle, both protective of established rights and exploring new arrangements (e.g., community living and supported employment).

A paper prepared for the Leadership Institute on Community Integration by Turnbull and Turnbull (1989) looks toward the future, contrasting what they call "traditional views" on a number of topics with what they call the "state-of-the-art." Tables 3.1 and 3.2 present these contrasts concerning perceptions of disability and family members' roles.

Table 3.1. Perceptions of disability

Traditional	State of the art
1. A person with a disability is a burden to the family and society.	1. A person with a disability is a valued and contributing member of the family and society.
2. Families are dysfunctional because of the burden created by the person.	2. Society and its reactions to and policies about families and disability can create dysfunctionality in families.
3. Families correctly have low expectations, particularly for segregated services and second-class citizenship, because it is unrealistic for them to expect generic service providers to be willing to provide integrated services.	3. Families should be supported to have high expectations for, and skills to obtain, integrated services and full citizenship.

(Adapted from Turnbull & Turnbull [1989], pp. 2–3.)

FAMILY SYSTEMS AND ADAPTATION

The family's role in the development of a child with disabilities has gained increasing attention, as well as changing focus. From an intensive focus on the development of the child, increasingly there is exploration of "the surrounding relationships within the family system" (Gallagher & Bristol, 1989, p. 295).

The sophistication and professionalization (perhaps to the point of overkill) of this new focus is seen in the following excerpt from a synopsis of the research design of a study, "Effects on families of children with a traumatic brain injury to be studied" (Nagle, 1989).

First, family system resources will be measured by the Olson, et al. (1985) FACES III (Family Adaptability and Cohesion Scales). As another measure of family system resources, McCubbin et al.'s (1983) CHIP (Coping-Health Inventory for Parents), as adapted by Brown and McCormack (1987), will be used to draw off of the family's capacity to solve effectively problems derived from the continuing care of the child with TBI. Second, Procidano and Heller's (1983) measure of perceived social support from friends and family will be used to operationalize social support. Third, family stressor pile-up will be measured by McCubbin, Patterson,

Table 3.2.   Family members' roles

Traditional	State of the art
1. Mothers are the family members who are the most interested in being involved in services for the child.	1. Every family should have the opportunity to designate the appropriate members to take on various roles in its and the person's life over the life span.
2. Parents of adults over-protect them; therefore, adults should be independent from their parents and rely upon professional family substitutes.	2. Adults with disabilities have the opportunity to identify and act on their preferences of the roles of their family, as well as the roles of others who may have significance in their lives.
3. Siblings (particularly sisters) should take responsibility for long-term care of their brother or sister, both before and after their parents' death.	3. Siblings, like parents, are entitled to normalization and to their own lives. It should not be automatically presumed that they will always be available to have a role with regard to their brother or sister.
4. When any family member is particularly severely "distressed" by the person with a disability, a "parentectomy" or other separation of the person from the family is warranted, with the person with a disability being placed outside of the family.	4. There are various appropriate means of supporting the family so that it is able to provide a supportive home to all members, including the person with a disability. Permanency planning, which means supporting the family and ensuring that the person with a disability has a wholesome family environment, is especially helpful.

(Adapted from Turnbull & Turnbull [1989], p. 5.)

and Wilson's (1980) FILE (Family Inventory of Life Events and Changes). As another measure of family stressor pile-up, Jacob's (1987) indices of skill proficiency in the areas of self-care, mobility, cognition, social and adaptive living, and communication will be used. Fourth, coherence and meaning will be operationalized by questionnaire items that will be fashioned to measure (a) the family's commitment to sustaining the child with TBI at home, (b) the degree to which family members feel they can predict the immediate future in terms of work and family, (c) the perceived "fit" between the family and its immediate environment. Fifth, family adaptation will be measured by Olson's (1982) satisfaction scale relating to the dimensions of family cohesion and adaptability as well as a family distress checklist of emotional, marital, health, financial, and legal problems the family may have needed to confront in the past three months. These two measures of family adaptation were predicated on the basic assumption that the continued survival of the family as a functional entity depends on its achieving an acceptable balance between family satisfaction and distress while meeting the needs of each family member. (p. 7)

And beyond this:

There are intergenerational factors influencing the parents' behaviors and roles. There are also the larger cultural groups to which the family owes loyalty, such as extended family and friends, the church, social clubs, and those social policies that influence the family system either directly or through the other systems with which the family comes in contact. (p. 295)

There are a variety of theoretical approaches to family studies, each emphasizing different dimensions of family functioning and dynamics. Florian (1989) identifies Kantor and Lehr's (1975) affect and power; Minuchin's (1974) enmeshment and disengagement; Moos's (1976) relationships, personal growth, and system maintenance; Beavers's (1977) closeness/autonomy and power negotiation; Riess's (1981) configuration, coordination, and closure; and Olson, Sprenkle, and Russell's (1979) circumplex model of three dimensions of family dynamics—family cohesion, family adaptability, and family communication.

Parsons and Bales (1955) distinguish between instrumental and expressive parental roles: instrumental roles are concerned with exercising control over the child while expressive roles are concerned with the emotional aspects of parenting, with control mediated through affection. Parents, including those of children with disabilities, need

to learn to cope with both the instrumental and expressive aspects of their roles if they are to contribute to the overall development of their child. Factors that affect the parents' ability to participate effectively in this socialization process include socio-economic status, age of parents, sex of children, birth order of child, religious orientation, parents' own status as a handicapped or non-handicapped person. (Parsons & Bales, 1955, pp. 48–49)

While most family development models have not incorpo-rated consideration of families with a child with disabilities, some have done so, including Belsky and Tolan (1981), Bron-fenbrenner (1977, 1979), Sameroff and Chandler (1975), and Thomas and Chess (1977). In describing the transactional model developed by Sameroff and Chandler and by Sameroff (1980), Fewell (1986) notes that it "reflects a link between risk factors and development outcome" (p. 4) that results "from a continual interplay between a changing child and a changing environment . . . " (Sameroff, 1980, p. 345). Fewell (1986) cites a number of studies that suggest that "the contribution of the impairment to the transactions between parent and child may be so strongly influenced by the impairment that this single factor accounts for the quality of the transactions between the parent and the child" (p. 5).

A contrary view, which we share, suggests "that no stressful event or stressor, including the presence or care of a handi-capped child, invariably causes a family crisis" (Gallagher & Bristol, 1989, p. 301). The findings of a study comparing the values mothers in Japan, Puerto Rico, and the United States mainland hold for their children reinforces this point, reporting that "the presence or absence of a handicap in the child did not have an overall effect upon the [culture-based] values held by the mothers for their preschoolers" (Quirk et al., 1986, p. 482).

Hill (1949, 1958) proposed a theory of family stress in which the characteristics of the stressor event (A), the family's internal crisis-meeting resources (B), and the family's defini-tion of the stressor (C) contribute to the prevention or pre-cipitation of family crisis (X). The ABCX model has been further developed to deal also with postcrisis adaptation. McCubbin and Patterson (1981, 1983) proposed a double ABCX model or Family Adjustment and Adaptation Response model (FAAR). To the original ABCX model, the Double ABCX model adds the pile-up of other family stressors which make adaptation more diffi-cult (aA); the social and psychological resources (bB), and cop-ing strategies (BC) which the family uses in managing potential crisis situations; the meaning the family assigns to the event (cC); and the range of both positive and negative outcomes possible. Gallagher and Bristol (1989) argue that the Double ABCX model is useful because it

> places emphasis on adaptation over time, is an ecological model which recognizes the social and contextual nature of adaptation over time, provides for assessment of active coping as well as passive support, *addresses the possibility that healthy adaptation rather than pathology may characterize the family's response to stress.* . . . [italics added] (p. 301)

Furthermore, they say that it has been empirically demonstrated to be applicable to adaptation in families with a child with disabilities.[4,5]

The most helpful coping strategies used by at least two-thirds of the families in the studies reported on by Gallagher and Bristol (1989) were (in decreasing order of helpfulness): believing that the child's intervention program had the family's best interest at heart, learning how to help their children improve, believing in God, talking over personal feelings and concerns with their spouses, building closer relationships with spouses, trying to maintain a stable family life, developing themselves as persons, telling themselves they had many things to be thankful for, doing things with their children, and believing that their children will get better. Among the least helpful were eating and allowing themselves to become angry (p. 305). Another major mediator of stress is the ideology or subjective beliefs (element C in the ABCX model) the family holds regarding having a child with disabilities.

---

[4]Among the more interesting findings from an extensive array of studies that Gallagher and Bristol (1989) report are: the ABCX model predicted healthy adaptation in families of children with developmental disabilities; family stress of adaptation varies as a function of the type of the child's handicap; among other specific child characteristics that have been related to better adaptation is child age, with parents of younger children expressing less stress than parents of older children; informal supports affect not only maternal feelings, but also the mother's interaction with the child with a disability; high quality, appropriate formal services can contribute not only to child gain but to successful family adaptation; inadequate or inappropriate services, however, may increase family stress.

[5]For additional reports on the use of the ABCX model, see Turnbull et al. (1986). For a more critical view of the ABCX regarding individuals, see Singer and Irvin (1989a).

In summary,[6] Gallagher and Bristol state:

> The majority of parents of young handicapped children, then,
> through the use of resources, active coping strategies, and sub-
> jective beliefs are able to mediate the stress of their child and
> adapt successfully to the very real demands of their difficult situa-
> tions. (p. 306)

LIFE CYCLE NEEDS

Not only are there differences among families in terms of coping
style and capacity, there are differences across the life cycle of
the child and the family (Fewell & Vadasy, 1986). Just as individuals change over time and have differing developmental
tasks across the life cycle, so do small groups, including couples and families (Olson et al., 1983). Turnbull and Turnbull
(1986) have related life cycle stages to common concerns that
relatives have about a family member with a disability. This
concept, combined with a broad understanding of family composition and dynamics, is the basis for the family systems approach (Turnbull, Brotherson, & Summers, 1985; Turnbull,
Turnbull, Bronicki, Summers, & Roeder-Gordon, 1989; Turnbull & Winton, 1984). A virtue of the approach is seeing "the
essential similarity in many respects between families of dis-

---

[6]There are two issues as to effects of a child with a disability on families that
we have not addressed. These are separation and divorce in families with a child
with disabilities and single-parent families. As to the first, after noting the
methodological problems, both in terms of sampling and distinguishing causes
from effects, Gallagher and Bristol (1989) state: "Our data indicate that if
samples are of adequate size and appropriate comparison samples are used,
families of at least some handicapped children, especially American families, are
at greater risk for marital break-down when their children are young, than are
families of young, nonhandicapped children" (p. 300). As to single-parent families, Gallagher and Bristol (1989) note that they make up a large segment of the
families of children with disabilities, citing a study "Of the 1,050 families
surveyed in a free, statewide program for developmentally disabled children,
41% were headed by a single-parent, including those who were separated, never
married or divorced" (p. 300). Bristol (in press) goes on to note that: blanket
assumptions regarding no father involvement in single-parent families and high
father involvement in two-parent families are misleading; persons other than
parents contribute significantly to child rearing in these families and should be
included in research and assessment descriptions of child rearing environments; research on single parents should control for type of single parenthood;
control for socioeconomic differences between two-parent and single-parent
families is critical in designing research and interpreting results; coping with
single parenthood is a process that changes and must be measured over time;
and the deficit model of "broken homes" is not useful or constructive.

abled children and families of non-disabled children. . . . In general, families meet the day to day problems created by the child's disability in ways that are fairly typical of the behaviour of any other family" (Mittler, Mittler, & McConachie, 1987, p. 18).

In effect, then, there are two entwined and interacting life cycles: that of the family as a unit and that of individual members, including the child with a disability. Something of the range of these cycles is seen in Singer and Irvin (1989b) about families with a child with a disability, which covers support for families during the child's infancy (Hanson, Ellis, & Deppe, 1989), early intervention (Slentz, Walker, & Bricker, 1989), support during the school years (Goetz, Anderson, & Laten, 1989), support in the transition from school to post-secondary activities (Halvorsen, Doering, Farron-Davis, Usilton, & Sailor, 1989), supported employment (Sowers, 1989), and planning for life after the parents' death (Apolloni, 1989). Another aspect concerns the consequences for and roles of siblings (Powell & Ogle, 1985; Skrtic, Summers, Brotherson, & Turnbull, 1984; Taylor, Knoll, Lehr, & Walker, 1989; Tinsley & Parke, 1984). While stages may be fixed, meaning is culturally loaded. Turnbull and Turnbull (1987) report on cultural traditions in Central and South America (and their meaning for policies concerning Latino students in United States schools). They contrast family traditions and then turn to their meaning in the process of transition from school to post-secondary activities for youth with disabilities. (See Table 3.3.) In terms of the transition process for youth with disabilities, Turnbull and Turnbull (1987) report that among Latino families it does not mean establishing a life independent of the family, or living separately from the family, or employment outside of the family's influence, or a social life outside of the family's network.

Roberts (1986) illustrates several life stages in a chapter describing the experiences of three mothers,[7] one with a new-

---

[7]Despite some changes, it is mothers who play the major role in child care, for children with or without disabilities. To the extent that for the former there are increased responsibilities, the mothers' burden is increased. Wilberta Donovan points out that this role differentiation not only is a fact in practice, it is embedded in the way research and studies are conducted. She notes, for example, that when the question is posed as to the father's contribution to a child's rearing, it is called "support," with the implication that child care is (and ought to be) the mother's responsibility (Research on parenting, 1988, pp. 9–10).

Table 3.3. Contrasting tendencies

United States	Latin America
Independence from parental family encouraged	Unity, permanence, and retention with family of origin expected
Nuclear family	Extended family
Protective but accelerate child's development	Protective, prolonging dependence
Family members independent	Family members interdependent
Use formal support systems	Use informal support systems before formal; prefer private to governmental, when formal support used
Individualism rewarded; development is primary goal of policy and service systems	Happiness more important than development
Competitive	Cooperative
Future oriented	Present oriented
Impermanent and transitory	Permanent

(Adapted from Turnbull & Turnbull [1987], p. 3.)

born, the other with a child in elementary school, and the third with an adolescent. While, of course, there are differing issues in each family, there are some common themes, including adjustment and readjustment, the cycles of emotion, information gathering, and the parent-professional relationship.

A unique "stage" is described by Lord and Farlow (1987), who report on the involvement of parents with their children who are "deinstitutionalized." Describing the process in British Columbia, Canada with the closing of Tranquille, a large institution for persons with developmental disabilities, they report:

> After years of accepting the decisions of professionals, and resigning themselves to the fact that they had very little input into their child's institutionalized life, a number of parents were provoked into action with the closure of the institution. (p. 26)

Parents who became involved identified four experiences which led to this change:

Attending parent meetings
Observing community living options

Participating with a mentor
Participating in individual program planning. (p. 29)

These individual activities were part of an organizational strategy that included:

A decentralized regional effort
A family support concept devised by British Columbians for Mentally Handicapped People
Regional resource developers, hired by the British Columbia Ministry of Human Resources, who were committed to family involvement. (p. 31)

PARENTAL INVOLVEMENT

Another way to address these issues is to consider the variety of roles that parents may play. Slentz, Walker, and Bricker (1989) identify the following roles: parents as advocates, parents as learners and interventionists, parents as recipients of services, and parents as decision-makers. Epstein (On parents and schools, 1989) presents a range of examples illustrating five types of parental involvement; they are shown in Table 3.4.

Beginning in the 1950s, parents increasingly began to advocate on behalf of their children: for keeping them out of institutions, for educational services (initially through parent-organized programs and then with PL 94-142 [the Education For All Handicapped Children Act, 1975] in the public schools), and currently for employment and community living programs. The extensive needs of some children with disabilities, and the often-held assumption that "inside every mother is an enthusiastic therapist with time on her hands" (Kaiser & Hayden, 1984, p. 304) have led to numerous efforts to engage parents as lay teachers or therapists with their children. Parents have now come to be seen as direct objects of services; while most of these programs have been for mothers, some serve fathers, and a few serve siblings or grandparents. Parents act as decision-makers both in terms of their own children, by the due process rights of PL 94-142, and sometimes at the program level as well. In considering any of these (and other) roles, it is important both to recognize that there are class and cultural differences in the extent to which parents have been successfully engaged in any

Table 3.4. Examples of practices to promote, and outcomes from, the five types of parent involvement

Type 1 Parenting	Type 2 Communicating	Type 3 Volunteering	Type 4 Learning at home	Type 5 Representing other parents
Help all families establish home environments to support learning	Design more effective forms of communication to reach parents	Recruit and organize parent help and support	Provide ideas to parents on how to help child at home	Recruit and train parent leaders

A few examples of practices of each type

Type 1 Parenting	Type 2 Communicating	Type 3 Volunteering	Type 4 Learning at home	Type 5 Representing other parents
School provides suggestions for home conditions that support learning at each grade level	Teachers conduct conferences with every parent at least once a year, with follow-up as needed	School volunteer program or class parent and committee of volunteers for each room	Information to parents on skills in each subject at each grade. Regular homework schedule (once a week or twice a month) that requires students to discuss schoolwork at home	Participation and leadership in PTA/PTO or other parent organizations, including advisory councils or committees such as curriculum, safety, and personnel
Workshops, videotapes, computerized phone messages on parenting and child-rearing issues at each grade level	Translators for language-minority families	Parent Room or Parent Club for volunteers and resources for parents	Calendars with daily topics for discussion by parents and students	Independent advocacy groups
	Weekly or monthly folders of student work are sent home and reviewed and comments returned	Annual postcard survey to identify all available talents, times, and locations of volunteers		

A few examples of outcomes linked to each type

Parent outcomes

Self-confidence in parenting	Understanding school programs	Interaction with child as student at home	Input to policies that affect child's education
Knowledge of child development	Interaction with teachers	Support and encouragement of schoolwork	Feeling control of environment
Understanding of home as environment for student learning	Monitoring child's progress	Participation in child's education	

Student outcomes

Security	Student participation in parent-teacher conferences, or in preparation for conferences	Homework completion	Rights protected
Respect for parent	Better decisions about courses, programs	Self-concept of ability as learner	Specific benefits linked to specific policies
Improved attendance		Achievement in skills practiced	
Awareness of importance of school		Ease of communication with adults	

Teacher outcomes

Understanding of family cultures, goals, talents, needs	Knowledge that family has common base of information for discussion of student problems, progress	Awareness of parent interest, in school and children, and willingness to help	Equal status interaction with parents to improve school programs
	Use of parent network for communications	Readiness to try programs that involve parents in many ways	Awareness of parent perspectives for policy development
		Respect and appreciation of parents' time, ability to follow through and reinforce learning	
		Better designs of homework assignments	

From: On parents and schools: A conversation with Joyce Epstein. (1989). *Educational Leadership, 47*(2), 26; reprinted with permission of the Association for Supervision and Curriculum Development. Copyright © 1989 by ASCD. All rights reserved.

of them,[8] and there is the preceding matter of whether a given parent should be obliged to play a particular role or any role.

Based upon research describing the impact of children with disabilities upon the family and reports of parents, Wiegerink and Comfort (1987) describe the needs of parents with a child with disabilities. The most frequently cited need is for accurate information regarding their child's diagnosis and prognosis. Practitioners are faulted for disregarding parents' concerns and for withholding information. In addition to information about their child's impairment, parents require information regarding the availability of services, and the ways to gain access to them. Once the program is located, parents need a clear explanation of its rationale, goals, and options for participation. For example, when a child enters a program, parents need to be regularly and accurately informed of the child's individual program and progress. Ongoing emotional support is needed by many parents, although its nature and character will vary. While some families will need assistance with routine activities of care and/or financial assistance, others will require few or no services.

While parental involvement has generally been hailed as desirable, there have been critiques of parental involvement activities, both in particular and conceptually. As Lipsky (1985) points out, much of the effort to involve parents is part of a deficit model, with professionals blaming parents for the ills of the child. Johnson and Chamberlin (1983) suggest that given the focus on weaknesses of parents, programs focus on training parents in how to teach, feed, or to manage child behavior, while little attention is given to other parent or family needs. Farber and Lewis (1975) argue that school systems have embraced parent involvement as a fad, both to reduce costs and to transfer responsibility for educational failure. Stevens (1978) expresses concern about the unanticipated detrimental effects on parents of inadequate or inappropriate programs, indicating that "haphazard programs may operate to shake the confi-

---

[8]A report on parental involvement in education in the United Kingdom reports class and racial group differences (Rogers, 1986). And a study of four school systems in the United States found that "a white, married mother who graduated from high school was 5.4 times more likely than a non-white, single mother who had not graduated from high school, to have attended the most recent IEP conference held for her child" (Singer & Butler, 1987, p. 146).

dence a parent has acquired . . . " (p. 64). And Rutherford and Edgar (1979) urge parental involvement in decision-making but not in day-to-day classroom activities, arguing that they need a respite from their responsibilities to a child with disabilities. Turnbull and Winton (1984) make a similar point, but rather than recommending parent involvement overall, they suggest that programs offer a variety of choices including the option of nonparticipation.

More fundamental than challenges to particular aspects of parent involvement programs is Wood's (1989) critique of parental involvement. She refers to Dessent's phrase, the "new philosophy of parentology" (p. 200), as the latest fad in education, and cites Pugh's (1987) report, from a study of parents' needs in United Kingdom preschools, that

> parents tended to feel confused and lacking in confidence in the face of professional expertise . . . made to feel that there must be a "right way" to bring children up if only they could decide which expert to believe. . . . They also think they should not try what they intuitively feel is right unless an "expert" has advised it. (p. 94)

Wood (1989) says that this new philosophy of parentology might be labeled as deskilling:

> The growth in the recognition of the importance of home life and pre-school years for the developing child and young adult appears to have brought with it a corresponding growth in the professionals needed to service this area. The home has not been a traditional site for intervention for educationalists, yet the social pathology model of special education needs offers the professionals the legitimate authority to implement pre-school home-based intervention, and the ideology of benevolent humanitarianism reinforces the intervention as a helpful extension of special education, professionals helping parents in partnership. (p. 201)

McKnight (1977) has pointed to the "disabling" help that characterizes much of professional interventions. Furthermore, Pugh (1987) has noted

> that making parents feel responsible for their children's successes, as in the Portage teaching model, also means making them feel responsible for their failures. Parents may see the child's performance as a measure of their own success. Such a model also makes it easy for the professionals to blame "uncooperative" "unmotivated" parents rather than examining their own methods and approaches.

> Individualizing need removes people and "their" difficulties from a social context and out of the political arena. Furthermore, clients are increasingly understood as a "set of manageable parts" each of which requires its own service mechanic. (p. 201)

Darling's (1979, 1988) conceptualization of the parent as entrepreneur addresses some of the criticism that Wood offers:

> Like the members of social movements and deviant sub-cultures, . . . parents come to redefine the world. . . . A child's birth defect cannot be changed; therefore, society must be changed or made responsive to the needs of the child and the child's family. Parents who have been socialized to love, nurture, and socialize their children have no choice but to become entrepreneurs in their own interest. Parental actions can thus be explained as readily in terms of social structure and social interaction as in terms of guilt or defense mechanism. (Darling, 1979, p. 223)

> Parents begin to take the initiative in promoting their child's cause as a result of repeated negative interactions with medical, education, and social agencies, each of which might serve as a critical turning point, combined with support from significant others. Organized associations of parents of children with similar problems play an important role here. [A]s parents become more closely integrated in proparent (and sometimes antiprofessional) networks, their commitment to entrepreneurial activities is likely to increase. (Darling, 1979, p. 225)

Increasingly, there is talk of a parent-professional partnership, as a way to recognize the respective roles. For some this is little more than the old asymmetry between professionals and parents in a new garb, and they have have put forward models of greater equality.

PARENT-PROFESSIONAL PARTNERSHIPS

Throughout this chapter we have noted ways in which parent-professional interactions have been harmful. Singer and Irvin (1989a) point out that "in the worst cases, parents have reported feeling intimidated, unheard, or dismissed by the professionals who are trying to help them" (p. 17). More fundamental is the recognition that some modes of helping can (inadvertently or not) reduce family members' ability to solve their own problems.

Fisher (1983) and other social

psychologists have explored the impact of helping relationships on recipients' perceptions of themselves and others. . . . Dunst and Trivette (in press) have expressed concern that traditional modes of assisting parents of handicapped infants may potentially induce helplessness. (Singer & Irvin, 1989a, p. 17)

McKnight (1977) sees disabling effects as intrinsic to modern professional services, because of the basic assumption that "you are the problem" and "I'm the professionalized servicer, and am the answer" (cited in Wood, 1989, p. 202).

Along the same line, Wood (1989) writes:

Seldom do professionals recognize that their expectation that parents *should* [italics in the original] cooperate with them is a value judgment, based on taken-for-granted assumptions about what it means to be a "good" parent. Rather, . . . professionals see parental cooperation as a means of enhancing their effectiveness and minimizing the child's learning difficulties. The expectation of parental involvement and partnership is viewed as stemming from professionals' own knowledge and expertise. (p. 203)

The issue goes beyond the behavior of individual professionals, or even professionals in general. The traditional pathological concepts of disability remain predominant in both professional practice and everyday life. As Tomlinson (1982) has pointed out, speaking about special education, although it is equally true about other services for persons with disabilities:

The rhetoric of special education needs draws attention to how to meet "recognized" needs and away from questioning why it is necessary for so many children to be categorized out of ordinary education in the first place. . . . (cited in Wood, 1989, p. 204)

Thus, Wood (1989) concludes:

Parent-professional partnership is something of a myth in its present terms even though individual relationships may be satisfying and empowering to both parties. If teachers want to consider partnership with parents in more depth they will have to be prepared to make themselves more aware of what special education is actually offering and why, of the processes they are involved in, whether intentionally or unintentionally, and the consequences for themselves, parents, and children. They will have to be prepared to alter structures to make room for parental choice, control, and evaluation. They will have to work in more open situations which involve sharing with and supporting other professionals, as well as parents. They will have to be prepared to critically examine their own practice themselves, and accept such from parents. They will have to be more open about what they are doing and why, to question their own motives, stances and the principles as well as the rhetoric upon which special education provision is based. (pp. 204–205)

While not entirely sanguine that such changes are likely to occur, we believe that there is reason to pursue the effort to form parent-professional partnerships (Lipsky, 1987). We do so, at least in part, because we believe that there is potential for success.

Parent-professional relationships have become a concern largely because of parents who have broken the quiet saint stereotype to articulate their need for services, and their desire not to be disenfranchised recipients of these services. (Healy, Keesee, & Smith, 1989, p. 43)

What needs to be worked through is the meaning, shape, and terms of the partnership. A comparison between traditional views of "partnership" and the state-of-the-art is presented by Turnbull and Turnbull (1989) in Table 3.5.

Mittler, Mittler, and McConachie (1987) cite recognition of the following factors as essential to a partnership.

1. Growth and learning in children can only be understood in relation to the various environments in which the child is living.
2. Parents and professionals concerned with the development of children with disabilities share a number of basic goals.
3. Parents and the extended family are the adults who are normally most accessible to the child.
4. Parents and professionals each have essential information which needs to be shared among all who are concerned with the child's development. (p. 5)

While parents and professionals each have essential information, as Mittler et al. (1987) point out, it is important to recognize that the desired partnership between parents and professionals must have at its base the understanding that parents and professionals are not alike. Also, is it not desirable for parents to become quasi-professionals; indeed, this seems the basis of many parent training programs. Not only does this perpetuate the deficit model that has been discussed earlier, it misconstrues the roles of the two parties, and their rela-

Table 3.5. Family-person-professional partnership

Traditional	State of the art
1. Professionals should formulate the person's and the parents' needs and the person and parents should at least acquiesce to and agree with the professionals' perspective. If they do not, they need "treatment" and are "pathological."	1. Families identify their own needs; the person identifies his or her own needs. They may choose to use or decline to use professional assistance from generic or specialized service-professionals to identify or satisfy their preferences and needs.
2. On the basis of their identification, professionals should prescribe how to satisfy the person's and the parents' needs and the person and parents should agree with the professionals' prescription or else risk being "diagnosed" as needing "treatment" for their "pathology."	2. Families and the person choose the degree to which they work with generic or specialized professionals and with the informal network to meet their needs and satisfy their preference.
3. Professionals should design formal service programs to meet the person's and parents' needs, and the person and parents should accept (participate in and appreciate) those programs.	3. Families and the person form a partnership with generic or specialized professionals in designing formal and informal service programs, choosing the degree to which they participate, and helping to modify programs to make them more responsive.
4. Professionals should set policies and design formal service systems to meet the person's needs, and parents should advocate for what professionals want.	4. Families and the person form a partnership with generic or specialized professionals in setting policy and designing the formal service system to meet their needs, and in advocating for responsive policy and systems.

(continued)

Table 3.5. (continued)

Traditional	State of the art
5. White, middle- and upper-class parents are the only ones willing and interested in attending individualized conferences and training workshops with professionals; it can be assumed, however, that these parents generally speak for all parents.	5. Many families characterized by racial or ethnic minority and lower socio-economic status have encountered system and individual barriers to establishing partnerships with professionals. Full accommodation should be made based on their preferences and needs, and it should be recognized that it most likely is erroneous to assume that white middle- and upper-class parents represent minority families' interests.

(Adapted from Turnbull & Turnbull [1989], pp. 7–8.)

tionships to the child.[9] Parents and professionals have different relationships to the child. The parents' relationship is individual, intimate, lifelong, and subjective. The professional's involvement with the child is time-delimited, in the context of many other children, and partakes of objectivity. Neither of these is better than the other; they are different. The expertise of parents and of professionals is equivalent. (A recognition of this would be the implementation of training programs for professionals conducted by parents, in addition to parent training programs conducted by "professionals," which already exist.) As with most partnerships, it is in bringing together persons with differing skills and aptitudes—differing expertise—that a successful relationship can be developed.

---

[9]Turnbull and Turnbull (1989) uniquely emphasize in Table 3.5 that the partnership must be three-way, including not only parents and professionals but also the individual with the disability. Given that our interest here is on families with young children, our focus is on the parent-professional partnership; however, it is essential that the infantalization that so often characterizes treatment of persons with disabilities not be perpetuated by their exclusion from a determining say in their own lives.

Effective partnerships rest on the basic recognition that both sides have areas of knowledge and skill that can contribute to the joint task of improving programs and services for the benefit of the child with disabilities. For this task, roles are complementary rather than separate and distinct. The partnership concept is built on professional accountability to the parents. It includes mutual respect, sharing in a common purpose, joint decision-making, sharing feelings, and flexibility and honesty in dealing with each other.

While discussing interaction between professionals and parents of young children with handicaps, Healy et al. (1989) offer guidance appropriate to the development of partnerships at all levels.

1. While parents with at-risk and disabled children may at times be parents in crisis, they are not disabled parents. They have capacities for creative problem solving and coping that professionals need to respect, promote, and encourage.
2. Parents and involved professionals may have widely differing perspectives, experiences, and goals for a particular at-risk or disabled child. The difficult process of sharing and learning to understand these differing perspectives is an important part of care for the child.
3. To foster independence and competence in families, and to make the most effective use of services, it is critical for parents and professionals to distinguish between times when professional participation is important for good decisions, and times when the parent is singularly competent to make decisions in the child's and family's best interest. Inappropriate dependence is encouraged when professionals make decisions that should be made by parents.
4. Finding the professional balance between promoting competence and independence in families, on the one hand, and providing needed expertise and emotional support on the other, is part of a developmental process. A particular kind of support at one time may, at a later time, promote inappropriate dependence.
5. The goals of a partnership and teamwork between parents and professionals are difficult ones. The easiest pattern is for the professional to adopt the traditional role of knowledgeable decision maker and the parents to adopt that of passive recipients. Changing these roles takes commitment by both parties.
6. Lack of time and discontinuity of personnel are important and very real barriers to effective parent-professional collaboration.

7. The professional needs to share large amounts of information, often of a technical nature, with the parents of special needs children. This process can be aided by appropriate translation of technical language, the provision of relevant written materials, open acknowledgment of unknowns, and direction to other service providers.

8. Professional collaboration with families who have very young special needs children has a very strong interpersonal component. Case management should allow professionals who have developed a rapport with a family to take more responsibility for working with that family, and should also ensure that every family has an advocate.

9. Parents and professionals need to be drawn into a problem-solving diagnostic process that leads to answers for questions such as "What should be done?" and "What should it be called?"

10. Articulate, active parents have brought the issues of parent decision making into the spotlight, but not many start their careers as "special needs" parents with the skills to make it happen. It is part of the professionals' job to help parents identify goals and develop resources within themselves and within the service community to achieve them. (pp. 63–64)

A SENSE OF IDENTITY

Perhaps more than anything else that parents can give, children need a sense that they are desired, loved as they are. Marsha Forest (in press) cites Alice Walker on this point: "The most important lesson of all [learned in my childhood was]: that I did not need to be perfect to be loved. That no one does."

Wright (1983) notes that in studies looking at the characteristics and behaviors of parents of well-adjusted children: "What does stand out from the many diagnostically insignificant variations is the parents' statement of the 'most important of all'—namely, conveying to the children in behavior and words that they are loved, respected, and wanted" (p. 288).

Describing a scene of his early childhood, Nolan (1987), after bitterly excoriating his mother for "His arms, his legs, his useless body" (p. 38), was told by her that she loved him as he was. He then writes, in his Baroque style:

> Dread-filled fretting marked Joseph Meehan's [Nolan's name for himself] scene that day, but that scene and that day looked out through his eyes for the rest of his life. Comfort came in child-like notions, his clumsy body was his, but molested by mother-love he looked lolling looks at his limbs and liked Joseph Meehan. (p. 38)

Rousso (1984) adds to the same point, speaking about her mother's response to the way she walked:

> She made numerous attempts over the years of my childhood to have me go for physical therapy and to practice walking more normally at home. I vehemently refused all her efforts. She could not understand why I would not walk straight. Now, I realize why. My disability [cerebral palsy], with my different walk and talk and my involuntary movements, having been with me all my life, was part of me, part of my identity. With these disability features, I felt complete and whole. My mother's attempt to change my walk, strange as it may seem, felt like an assault on myself, an incomplete acceptance of all of me, an attempt to make me over. (p. 9)

Reflecting on this same dilemma from a parent's point of view, Park (1983) writes:

> Jessy [who has autism] can keep her reactions under control. Yet we have not wished completely to bid farewell to these strange products of the imagination, especially as in their absence her conversation is flatly factual, limited, and uninteresting. One does not wish to encourage "bizarre thinking," yet to discourage it entirely is to sacrifice much of the individuality and charm which are among her greatest assets. In the adolescent years, however, it had to be discouraged since it led so often to behavior too bizarre to be tolerated in the social world she was increasingly able to enter. (p. 286)

There is tension, then, in the effort of persons with disabilities to think of themselves in ways that incorporate their disability as an important part of their personal and social identity (Johnson, 1987). In the context of arguing for integration, Asch (in Ferguson & Asch, 1989) says:

> We do not want the point of integration to be a message such as that one young woman expressed about living with her family and being the only disabled student in her school: "I knew that I was all right because I was their daughter and they loved me, but my parents feel that blindness has icky consequences and [they] don't like other blind people and don't want me to know them." And another young disabled man recently commented how critical it was to meet other adults with his disability that he could like and respect. We do not want to create a new generation of students who repeat the mistakes of all too many disabled people who see themselves as "exceptions," who see disability as embarrassing, shameful, pitiable, but see themselves as unusually talented because they have achieved social or professional status within the nondisabled world. (p. 135)

Parents of a child with deafness (Spradley & Spradley, 1978) reflect on the same concern.

> We knew that Lynn would need more than our words and love. At first we found it painful to admit that we could not give Lynn all she needed to live in a hearing world. She needed the example of people like herself who had faced the same problems she would and solved them. Even at the age of six, Lynn had begun to see the world from the distinct perspective of her deafness. We could not entirely share that perspective. Bill and Bunny and other deaf friends could. Slowly we accepted the fact that only deaf people could provide *some* [italics added] things Lynn would need, helping her through *some* [italics added] of the important stages of childhood, pointing the way to a meaningful life. (p. 258).

There is increasing literature about the culture of disability, particularly within the community of persons with deafness (cf. Lane, 1984), but increasingly within the broader ambit of disability as a whole (cf. Hahn, 1987, 1988, 1989; Longmore, 1987; Zola, 1985; see also *Disability Rag*). An aspect of this is shown in the report of the first national survey of the attitudes of persons with disabilities (Harris & Associates, 1986). It reports that a plurality of persons surveyed feel that they "are a minority group in the same sense as are blacks and Hispanics" (p. 114). This is particularly true among those who are younger and those who have been disabled from birth.

Hahn (1989) offers the salient observation, particularly pertinent in the context of our concern about children with disabilities and their families, that

> unlike many minorities, persons with disabilities lack a feeling of generational continuity. If they acquire their disabilities as children, they are usually raised by nondisabled parents who might not be adequately prepared to provide a source of solace and understanding when their children encounter the animosity and aversion of the outside world. (p. 232)

Building on this point, Hahn (1989) points out that persons with disabilities share many experiences that may eventually become the basis of a distinctive subculture. Among these factors, he includes: "their almost universal exposure to the medical model [which leads] a disproportionate number of individuals with disabilities [to] become involved in a problematic relationship with physicians and professional authorities who seem to exercise undue influence over their personal activities"[10] (p. 232); the need for detailed planning to meet the routine demands of everyday life; the nature of the discrimination directed against the minority of disabled persons, which he attributes either to an "existential" anxiety, the worry that "there but by the grace of God go I," or to an "aesthetic" anxiety—the fearful response to others whose appearance is perceived as unpleasant or upsetting. He emphasizes this latter point, stating:

> Aversion to persons with disabilities could be a principle explanation for the failure of the disabled minority to develop a positive sense of personal and political identity. The development of such an identity is an essential foundation of the movement to improve the status of persons with disabilities in society. Many men and women with disabilities are affected by the stigma that is also the major source of their oppression. To be disabled not only involves functioning in an environment replete with obstacles that eventually may be circumvented or surmounted, but it also means living with a prominent physical characteristic that is generally considered unattractive. (p. 232–233)

An effort to bridge the lack of "generational continuity" is bringing together parents of children with disabilities with adults with disabilities, be they parents or not. "Through the Looking Glass," a program in Berkeley, California that provides services to parents who themselves are disabled, incorporates involvement of nondisabled parents of children with disabilities with adults with disabilities to allow the former to see in the latter the future of their own children, and the ways

---

[10]A Swedish writer with physical handicaps provides insight into what it means to be dependent upon others for the most private of functions:

> Few people are forced to expose themselves in the nude so often as the physically disabled who can't look after their own hygiene. Depersonalized into organic bundles, their bodies and private parts are washed. Erotic fantasies whirl around in the head like overheated spinning-tops when the nurse touches the erogenous zones between the legs or gives an enema. Your private parts are as depersonalized as yourself, they are washed and cleansed in a way regarded as natural for sick people; perhaps it is right, but the sexually deprived are forced to lie there exposed with expressionless faces, hoping that no-one will notice what pleasure or disgust they are experiencing. It is especially degrading for men [sic] to be aroused time and time again, to an unbearable point, only to be left in the certain knowledge that it will never be any different from this. (Enby cited in Craft & Craft, 1979, p. 12)

Some of this experience is shown in the film *My Left Foot*, portraying the life of Irish writer and painter Christy Brown.

adults cope with the realities of their disabilities (Kirshen-baum, 1985). In effect, it appropriately presents the adults with disabilities as experts. At the organizational level, in the United States the National Federation of the Blind has established a Parents of Blind Children Division, which includes among its activities encouraging these parents to come to the Federation's conventions and other activities to learn about the concerns and triumphs the current generation of adults with blindness experiences. Of course, among parents are persons with disabilities (Browne, Connors, & Stern, 1985). Whitman and Accardo (1990) address the topic of persons with mental retardation becoming parents, asking whether this is not "a logical, not unexpected, and not entirely undesirable outcome of normalization" (p. 205), while raising issues of a broader compass:

> In the absence of a commitment from society to provide an intensity of support services for parents who have mild to moderate mental retardation, the rights of children to a minimal expected parenting competence may need to severely restrict the rights of parents with mental retardation. If adequate parenting is a child's right, it becomes an adult's duty. (p. 9)

Exactly where and how to strike the balance in developing a positive sense of identity among children with disabilities is a complex matter. Ferguson (in Ferguson & Asch, 1989) does so as follows:

> For us, the approach is to begin with the natural setting and make sure Ian is included. Within that setting, it is not only appropriate, but beneficial, for Ian to have both disabled and nondisabled friends. I am not sure what Ian's sense of identity is, but I hope it includes an awareness at some level that his way of interacting with the world is not only acceptable, it is also *not* [italics in the original] unique. There are other people in wheelchairs; there are other people who do not talk well; there are other people who need a lot of help from others; there are, in short, other people like himself. (p. 136)

CONCLUSION

It is in keeping with our perspective to end this chapter with the focus on the child with a disability, and to emphasize both the child's uniqueness and commonness, her or his oneness with both persons with disabilities and persons who do not have disabilities. Also, it is in keeping with our views to end

with a focus on friends. While we have given considerable attention to family involvement with professionals, we recognize that
such relationships are—or at least should be—only a small
part of the child's (and family's) life. Too much of the lives of
persons with disabilities is professionalized, especially through
a medical perspective. Family and friends, kith and kin in the
language of the anthropologists, are both means and ends in
the lives of full participation that we seek.

Describing what professionals have learned from families,
Vincent (1988) says:

> Families are succeeding because they are able to build support
> networks which they can call upon when their individual re-
> sources are not enough to solve their problems. Parents are most
> likely to rely upon family members, friends, neighbors or cowork-
> ers for support when confronting problems in raising their chil-
> dren. Only as a last resort do they consult professionals. The
> implication of this finding for us is that we need to focus more of
> our attention in helping families develop and strengthen their
> own support networks. We need to emphasize to families that
> they are the ones best able to solve their own problems.
> Parents do need us, but not in the way we think they need us.
> They need us to do our job by making sure that our programs are
> the best possible, by providing help in a consistent way so they will
> not have to spend precious time in monitoring us closely. (p. 4)

In Chapters 4–9, we examine different aspects of supports
for families with a child with a disability. While any template or
organizational scheme is arbitrary and imposes upon the phenomena, we sought to design one that allowed unfettered consideration of the developments in each of the nine countries represented at the conference out of which this book grew, while
providing a common frame of reference for comparisons.

REFERENCES

Apolloni, T. (1989). Guardianship, trusts, and protective services. In
    G.H.S. Singer & L.K. Irvin (Eds.), *Support for caregiving families:
    Enabling positive adaptation to disability* (pp. 283–296). Bal-
    timore: Paul H. Brookes Publishing Co.
Beavers, W. (1977). *Psychotherapy and growth: A family systems per-
    spective.* New York: Bruner/Mazel.
Belsky, J., & Tolan, W.J. (1981). Infants as producers of their own
    development: An ecological analysis. In R.M. Lerner & N.A. Busch-

Rossnagel (Eds.), *Individuals as producers of their development* (pp. 87–115). New York: Academic Press.

Bristol, M.M. (in press). The home-care of developmentally disabled children: Some empirical support for a conceptual model of successful coping with family stress. In P. Vietze & S. Landesman-Dwyer (Eds.), *Living with retarded people. Monographs of the American Association on Mental Retardation.* Washington, DC: American Association on Mental Retardation.

Bronfenbrenner, U. (1977). Toward an experimental ecology of human development. *American Psychologist, 32,* 513–531.

Bronfenbrenner, U. (1979). *The ecology of human development: Experiments.* Cambridge, MA: Harvard University Press.

Brown, B.W., & McCormack, T. (1987, December). *Successful family coping in response to head injury.* National Head Injury Foundation 6th Annual Symposium, San Diego.

Browne, S., Connors, D., & Stern, N. (1985). *With the power of each breath.* Pittsburgh: Cleis Press.

Craft, A., & Craft, M. (1979). *Handicapped married couples: A Welsh study of couples handicapped from birth by mental, physical or personality disorder.* Boston: Routledge & Kegan Paul.

Darling, R. (1979). *Families against society: A study of reactions to children with birth defects.* Beverly Hills: Sage.

Darling, R.J. (1988). Parental entrepreneurship: A consumerist response to professional dominance. *Journal of Social Issues, 44*(1), 141–158.

Disability and the family: Life-style, not life-sentence. (1989). *Families and Disability Newsletter, I*(1), 1.

Dunst, C.J., & Trivette, C.M. (in press). Helping, helplessness, and harm. In J. Witt, S. Elliott, & F. Gresham (Eds.), *Handbook of behavior therapy in education.* New York: Plenum.

Ehlers, W.H. (1966). *The mothers of retarded children: How they feel; where they find help.* Springfield, IL: Charles C Thomas.

Farber, B., & Lewis, M. (1975). The symbolic use of parents: A sociological critique of educational practice. *Journal of Research and Development in Education, 8,* 34–43.

Ferguson, P.M., & Asch, A. (1989). What we want for our children: Perspectives of parents and adults with disabilities. In D. Biklen, D. Ferguson, & A. Ford (Eds.), *Schooling and disability* (pp. 108–140). Chicago: The University of Chicago Press.

Ferguson, P.M., & Ferguson, D. (1987). Parents and professionals. In P. Knoblock (Ed.), *Introduction to special education* (pp. 181–203). Boston: Little, Brown.

Fewell, R.R. (1986). A handicapped child in the family. In R.R. Fewell & P.F. Vadasy (Eds.), *Families of handicapped children: Needs and supports across the life span* (pp. 3–34). Austin: Pro-Ed.

Fewell, R.R., & Vadasy, P.F. (1986). *Families of handicapped children: Needs and supports across the life span.* Austin: Pro-Ed.

Fisher, J.D. (1983). Recipient reactions to aid: The parameters of the field. In J.D. Fisher, A. Nadler, & B.M. DePaulo (Eds.), *New direc-*

tions in helping: Vol. I. Recipient reactions to aid. New York: Academic Press.

Florian, V. (1989). The cultural impact on the family dynamics of parents who have a child with a disability. *Journal of Comparative Family Studies, 20*(1), 97–111.

Forest, M. (in press). It's about relationships. In L. Meyer, C. Peck, & L. Brown (Eds.), *Critical issues in the lives of persons with severe disabilities.* Baltimore: Paul H. Brookes Publishing Co.

Gallagher, J.J. (1956). Rejecting parents? *Exceptional Children, 22,* 273–276.

Gallagher, J.J., & Bristol, M. (1989). In M.C. Wang, M.C. Reynolds, & H.J. Walberg (Eds.), *Handbook of special education research and practice, Vol. 3: Low incidence conditions* (pp. 295–317). New York: Pergamon.

Gallagher, J.J., Scharfman, W., & Bristol, M. (1984). The division of responsibilities in families with preschool handicapped and nonhandicapped children. *Journal of Division for Early Childhood, 3,* 3–14.

Gliedman, J., & Roth, W. (1980). *The unexpected minority.* New York: Harcourt Brace Jovanovich.

Goetz, L., Anderson, J., & Laten, S. (1989). Facilitation of family support through public school programs. In G.H.S. Singer & L.K. Irvin (Eds.), *Support for caregiving families: Enabling positive adaptation to disability* (pp. 239–251). Baltimore: Paul H. Brookes Publishing Co.

Hahn, H. (1987). Civil rights for disabled Americans: The foundation of a political agenda. In A. Gartner & T. Joe (Eds.), *Images of the disabled/disabling images* (pp. 181–204). New York: Praeger.

Hahn, H. (1988). Can disability be beautiful? *Social Policy, 119* (3), 26–32.

Hahn, H. (1989). The politics of special education. In D.K. Lipsky & A. Gartner (Eds.), *Beyond separate education: Quality education for all* (pp. 225–242). Baltimore: Paul H. Brookes Publishing Co.

Halvorsen, A.T., Doering, K., Farron-Davis, F., Usilton, R., & Sailor, W. (1989). The role of parents and family members in planning severely disabled students' transitions from school. In G.H.S. Singer & L.K. Irvin (Eds.), *Support for caregiving families: Enabling positive adaptation to disbility* (pp. 253–268). Baltimore: Paul H. Brookes Publishing Co.

Hanson, M., Ellis, L., & Deppe, J. (1989). Support for families during infancy. In G.H.S. Singer & L.K. Irvin (Eds.), *Support for caregiving families: Enabling positive adaptation to disability* (pp. 207–219). Baltimore: Paul H. Brookes Publishing Co.

Harris & Associates. (1986). *The ICD survey of disabled Americans: Bringing disabled Americans into the mainstream.* New York: Author.

Healy, A., Keesee, P.D., & Smith, B.S. (1989). *Early services for children with special needs: Transactions for family support* (2nd ed). Baltimore: Paul H. Brookes Publishing Co.

Hill, R. (1949). *Families under stress: Adjustment to the crisis of war and separation.* New York: Harper & Row.

Hill, R. (1958). Social stress in the family. *Social Casework, 39,* 139–150.

Johnson, M. (1987, January/February). Emotion and pride. *Disability Rag, 3,*10.

Johnson, N.M., & Chamberlin, H.R. (1983). Early intervention: The state of the art. In *Developmental handicaps: Prevention and treatment* (pp. 1–23). Washington, DC: American Association of University Affiliated Programs for Persons with Developmental Disabilities.

Kagan, S.L., Powell, D.R., Weissbourd, B., & Zigler, E.F. (1987). *America's family support programs: Perspectives and prospects.* New Haven: Yale University Press.

Kaiser, C., & Hayden, A. (1984). Clinical research and policy issues in parenting severely handicapped infants. In J. Blacher (Ed.), *Severely handicapped young children and their families: Research in review* (pp. 275–318). Orlando: Academic Press.

Kanner, L. (1964). *A History of the care and study of the mentally retarded.* Springfield, IL: Charles C Thomas.

Kantor, D., & Lehr, W. (1975). *Inside the family.* San Francisco: Jossey-Bass.

Kaufman, S.Z. (1988). *Retarded isn't stupid, mom!* Baltimore: Paul H. Brookes Publishing Co.

Kellerman, S. (1989). Presentation at TASH Conference, Hunter College, New York City, January 21.

Kelly, J. (1989, July 1). When a child is seriously ill. *New York Newsday,* pp. II, 1–2.

Kirshenbaum, M. (1985). The disabled parent. In L. Aurenshine & H. Fenriquiez (Eds.), *Maternity nursing: Dimensions of change.* Belmont, CA: Wadsworth Press.

Lane, H. (1984). *When the mind hears: A history of the deaf.* New York: Random House.

Lehr, S. (1987, September). Family support . . . or is it ? *The Center on Human Policy Newsletter,* p. 3.

Lipsky, D.K. (1985). A parental perspective on stress and coping. *American Journal of Orthopsychiatry, 55*(4), 614–617.

Lipsky, D.K. (1987). *Family supports for families with a disabled member.* Monograph No. 39. New York: World Rehabilitation Fund.

Lipsky, D.K. (1989). The roles of parents. In D.K. Lipsky & A. Gartner (Eds.), *Beyond separate education: Quality education for all* (pp. 159–180). Baltimore: Paul H. Brookes Publishing Co.

Longmore, P. (1987). Uncovering the hidden history of people with disabilities. *Reviews in American History,* (September), 355–364.

Lord, J., & Farlow, D.M. (1987). Families and empowerment: A new dynamic in desinstitutionalization. *Entourage, 2*(4), 26–34.

Lusthaus, E. (n.d.). *Parental response to their children with mental disabilities: Reinterpreting the negative assumptions.* Unpublished manuscript.

MacKinnon, L., & Marlett, N. (1984). A social action perspective: The disabled and their families in context. In E.I. Coppersmith (Ed.), *Families with handicapped members* (pp. 111–126). Rockville, MD: Aspen Systems Corporation.

McCubbin, H.I., & Patterson, J. (1981). *Systematic assessment of family stress, resources and coping.* St. Paul: Family Stress Project, University of Minnesota.

McCubbin, H.I., & Patterson, J. (1983). Family adaptation to crises. In H.I. McCubbin, A. Cauble, & J. Patterson (Eds.), *Family stress, coping, and social support.* Springfield, IL: Charles C Thomas.

McDonald, E.T. (1979). Understand those feelings. In R.L. Noland (Ed.), *Counseling parents of the ill and the handicapped* (pp. 44–51). Springfield, IL: Charles C Thomas.

McKnight, J. (1977). Professional service and disabling help. In A. Brechin, P. Liddiard, & J. Swain (Eds.), *Handicap in social world.* London: Open University Press.

Minuchin, S. (1974). *Family and family therapy.* Cambridge, MA: Harvard University Press.

Mittler, P., Mittler, H., & McConachie, H. (1987). Family supports in England. In D.K. Lipsky (Ed.), *Family supports for families with a disabled member* (pp. 15–36). New York: World Rehabilitation Fund.

Moos, R. (1976). *The human context: Environmental determinants of behaviour.* New York: John Wiley & Sons.

Nagle, T.K. (1989). Effects on families of children with a traumatic brain injury to be satisfied. *NARIC Quarterly, 2*(1), 1, 6–8.

National Society for Children and Adults with Autism. (1981). *Help-children and families.* Washington, DC: Author.

Nolan, C. (1987). *Under the eye of the clock.* New York: Delta Publishing.

Olson, D.H., McCubbin, H.I., Barnes, H.L., Larsen, A.S., Muxen, M.J., & Wilson, M.A. (1983). *Families: What makes them work.* Beverly Hills: Sage Publications.

Olson, D.H., Sprenkle, D.H., & Russell, C.S. (1979). Circumplex model of marital and family systems: Cohesion and adaptability functions, family types, and clinical applications. *Family Process, 18*(1), 3–27.

On parents and schools: A conversation with Joyce Epstein. (1989). *Educational Leadership, 47*(2), 24–27.

Park, C.C. (1983). Growing out of autism. In E. Schopler & G.B. Mesibov (Eds.), *Autism in adolescents and adults.* New York: Plenum Press.

Parsons, T., & Bales, R.F. (1955). *Family socialization and interaction process.* New York: Free Press.

Pieper, E. (n.d.). *Sticks and stones: The story of loving a child.* Syracuse: Human Policy Press.

Powell, T.H., & Ogle, P.A. (1985). *Brothers and sisters: A special part of exceptional families.* Baltimore: Paul H. Brookes Publishing Co.

Procidano, M.E., & Heller, K. (1983). Measures of perceived social support from friends and from family: Three validation studies. *American Journal of Community Psychology, 11,* 1–24.

Pugh, G. (1987). Portage in perspective: Parental involvement in pre-school programmes. In R. Hedderly & K. Jennings (Eds.), *Extending and developing portage.* Windsor, UK: NFER-Nelson.

Quirk, M., Ciottone, R., Ninami, H., Wapner, S., Yammoto, T., Ishii, S., Lucca-Iriznay, P., & Pacheco, A. (1986). Values mothers hold for handicapped and nonhandicapped preschool children in Japan, Puerto Rico, and the US mainland. *International Journal of Psychology, 21,* 463–485.

Reid, E.S. (1979). Helping parents of handicapped children. In R.L. Noland (Ed.), *Counseling parents of the ill and the handicapped* (pp. 52–61). Springfield, IL: Charles C Thomas.

Research on parenting: Are scientists asking the right questions? (1988, Spring/Summer). *Family Support Bulletin,* p. 11–12.

Riess, D. (1981). *The family's construct of reality.* Cambridge, MA: Harvard University Press.

Roberts, M. (1986). Three mothers: Life-span experiences. In R.R. Fewell & P.F. Vadasy (Eds.), *Families of handicapped children: Needs and supports across the life span* (pp. 193–220). Austin: Pro-Ed.

Rogers, R. (1986). *Caught in the act: What LEAs tell parents under the 1981 Education Act.* London: Centre for Studies on Integration in Education.

Rothman, D. (1971). *The discovery of the asylum: Social order and disorder in the New Republic.* Boston: Little, Brown.

Rousso, H. (1984). Fostering healthy self-esteem. *Exceptional Parent, 9,* 9–11.

Routberg, M. (1986). *On becoming a special parent.* Chicago: Parent/Professional Publications.

Rubenstein, C. (1989, October 8). The baby bomb. *New York Times,* Part 2, pp. 34–38.

Rutherford, R.B., & Edgar, E. (1979). *Teachers and parents: A guide to interaction and cooperation.* Boston: Allyn & Bacon.

Sabbeth, B., & Leventhal, J.M. (1984). Marital adjustment to chronic childhood illness: A critique of the literature. *Pediatrics, 73*(6), 762–768.

Sameroff, A.J. (1980). Issues in early reproductive and caretaking risk: Review and current status. In D.B. Sawin, R.C. Hawkins, L.O. Walker, & J.H. Penticuff (Eds.), *Exceptional infant* (Vol. 4, pp. 343–359). New York: Brunner/Mazel.

Sameroff, A.J., & Chandler, M.J. (1975). Reproductive risk and the continuum of caretaking casualty. In F. Horowitz (Ed.), *Review of child development research* (pp. 187–243). Chicago: University of Chicago Press.

Sarason, S., & Doris, J. (1979). *Educational handicap, public policy, and social history.* New York: Free Press.

Schleifer, M.J., & Klein, S.D. (1985). *The disabled child and the family: An exceptional parent reader.* Boston: The Exceptional Parent Press.

Simons, R. (1987). *After the tears: Parents talk about raising a child with a disability.* New York: Harcourt Brace Jovanovich.

Singer, J.D., & Butler, J.A. (1987). The Education for All Handicapped Children Act: Schools as agents of social reform. *Harvard Educational Review, 57*(2), 125–152.

Singer, G.H.S., & Irvin, L.K. (1989a). Family caregiving, stress, and support. In G.H.S. Singer & L.K. Irvin, *Support for caregiving families: Enabling positive adaptation to disability* (pp. 3–25). Baltimore: Paul H. Brookes Publishing Co.

Singer, G.H.S., & Irvin, L.K. (1989b). *Support for caregiving families: Enabling positive adaptation to disability.* Baltimore: Paul H. Brookes Publishing Co.

Skrtic, T.M., Summers, J.A., Brotherson, M.J., & Turnbull, A.P. (1984). Severely handicapped children and their brothers and sisters. In J. Blacher (Ed.), *Severely handicapped young children and their families: Research in review* (pp. 215–246). New York: Academic Press.

Slentz, K.L., Walker, B., & Bricker, D. (1989). Supporting parent involvement in early intervention: A role-taking model. In G.H.S. Singer & L.K. Irvin (Eds.), *Support for caregiving families: Enabling positive adaptation to disability* (pp. 221–238). Baltimore: Paul H. Brookes Publishing Co.

Sowers, J. (1989). Critical parent roles in supported employment. In G.H.S. Singer & L.K. Irvin (Eds.), *Support for caregiving families: Enabling positive adaptation to disability* (pp. 269–282). Baltimore: Paul H. Brookes Publishing Co.

Spradley, T.S., & Spradley, J.P. (1978). *Deaf like me.* New York: Random House.

Stevens, J.H. (1978). Parent education programs: What determines effectiveness? *Young Children, 33,* 59–65.

Summers, J.A., Behr, S.K., & Turnbull, A.P. (1989). Positive adaptation and coping strengths of families who have children with disabilities. In G.H.S. Singer & L.K. Irvin (Eds.), *Support for caregiving families: Enabling positive adaptation to disability* (pp. 27–40). Baltimore: Paul H. Brookes Publishing Co.

Taylor, S.J., Knoll, J.A., Lehr, S., & Walker, P.M. (1989). Families for all children: Value-based services for children with disabilities and their families. In G.H.S. Singer & L.K. Irvin (Eds.), *Support for caregiving families: Enabling positive adaptation to disability* (pp. 41–53). Baltimore: Paul H. Brookes Publishing Co.

Thomas, A., & Chess, S. (1977). *Temperament and development.* New York: Brunner/Mazel.

Tinsley, B.R., & Parke, R.D. (1984). Grandparents as support and socialization agents. In M. Lewis (Ed.), *Beyond the dyad* (pp. 161–194). New York: Plenum.

Tomlinson, S. (1982). *A sociology of special education.* London: RKP.

Turnbull, A.P., Brotherson, M.J., & Summers, J.A. (1985). The impact of deinstitutionalization on families: A family systems approach. In R.H. Bruininks & K.C. Lakin (Eds.), *Living and learning in the least restrictive environment* (pp. 115–140). Baltimore: Paul H. Brookes Publishing Co.

Turnbull, H.R., Guess, D., & Turnbull, A.P. (1988). Vox Populi and Baby Doe. *Mental Retardation, 26*(3), 127–132.

Turnbull, A.P., Summers, J.A., Backus, L., Bronicki, G.J., Goodfriend, S.J., & Roeder-Gordon, C. (1986). *Stress and coping in families having a member with a developmental disability.* Washington, DC: D:ATA Institute.

Turnbull, A.P., & Turnbull, H.R. (Eds.). (1978). *Parents speak out: Growing with a handicapped child.* Columbus: Charles E. Merrill.

Turnbull, A.P., & Turnbull, H.R. (1986). *Families, professionals, and exceptionality: A special partnership.* Columbus: Charles E. Merrill.

Turnbull, H.R., & Turnbull, A.P. (1987). *The Latino family and public policy in the United States: Informal support and transition into adulthood.* New York: World Rehabilitation Fund.

Turnbull, A.P., & Turnbull, H.R. (1989). Families and community integration. In *Proceedings: Leadership Institute on Community Integration.* Syracuse, NY: Center on Human Policy.

Turnbull, H.R., Turnbull, A.P., Bronicki, G.J., Summers, J.A., & Roeder-Gordon, C. (1989). *Disability and the family: A guide to decisions for adulthood.* Baltimore: Paul H. Brookes Publishing Co.

Turnbull, A.P., & Winton, P.J. (1984). Parent involvement policy and practice: Current research and implications for families of young, severely handicapped children. In J. Blacher (Ed.), *Severely handicapped young children and their families: Research in review* (pp. 377–400). New York: Academic Press.

Vance, J.C., Fazan, L.E., Satterwhite, B., & Pless, I.B. (1980). Effects of nephrotic syndrome on the family: A controlled study. *Pediatrics, 64*, 948–955.

Vincent, L.J. (1988). What we have learned from families. *Family Support Bulletin,* (Fall), 3.

Walker, B. (1989). Stategies for improving parent-professional cooperation. In G.H.S. Singer & L.K. Irvin (Eds.), *Support for caregiving families: Enabling positive adaptation to disability* (pp. 103–120). Baltimore: Paul H. Brookes Publishing Co.

Whitman, B.Y., & Accardo, P.J. (1990). *When a parent is mentally retarded.* Baltimore: Paul H. Brookes Publishing Co.

Wiegerink, R., & Comfort, M. (1987). Parent involvement: Support for families of children with special needs. In S.L. Kagan, D.R. Powell, B. Weissbourd, & E.F. Zigler (Eds.), *America's family support programs: Perspectives and prospects.* New Haven: Yale University Press.

Wright, B.A. (1983). *Physical disability: A psychological approach.* New York: Harper & Row.

Wood, S. (1989). Parents: Whose partners? In L. Baxton (Ed.), *The politics of special education needs* (pp. 190–207). London: The Falmer Press.

Zola, I.K. (1985). Depictions of disability—Metaphor, message, and medium in the media: A research and political agenda. *The Social Science Journal, 22*(4), 5–17.

4

Basic Social Welfare Provisions and Financial Assistance

Among the nine countries there is a considerable range in basic social welfare arrangements, from the rich array of public sector provisions in Sweden to Kenya's limited resources, from the United States' reliance upon employment-based benefits to Canada's increasing socialization of "natural" networks. Along a different axis, there is variety among the countries as to the extent that services for persons with disabilities are an integral part of the general social welfare system. For example, in Sweden there is considerable overlap with the general social welfare system, in contrast with the United States where a quite separate system serves persons with disabilities. And, of course, the type and amount of assistance provided is widely different in the nine countries.[1]

Arrangements for financial assistance also vary among the countries. They can be viewed in two aspects: 1) who is eligible for financial assistance and 2) the type of assistance provided. As to eligibility for government-provided assistance, there is division according to countries that

[1] For an excellent analysis of social security disability programs across several countries, including three that are a part of our study, see Duncan and Woods (1987).

Provide assistance to all children
Provide assistance to all children with disabilities
Provide assistance to some children depending upon family
    income (or social circumstance)
Provide assistance to some children with disabilities
    depending upon family income (or social circumstance)

Implicit here is the distinction between the general provision of services for all children, or all those with special needs, as part of a general social welfare scheme, versus particular services dependent upon a category of need (especially income, i.e., means-tested benefits) or conditions. Of the nine countries reviewed, only Sweden and Australia provide assistance to all children, without family income requirements.

A similar division applies to support for families. Only Sweden provides support to all families with a child with a disability. Each of the other countries to some extent provides support to some families, with some countries including families with a child with a disability. Where support is provided to children with disabilities (or to their families), most often that support varies by both the nature (or category) of the child's impairment, as well as its severity. Sweden provides support for all families regardless of whether the child has a disability.

The types of assistance provided also vary widely among the countries. They include:

Direct cash payments
Direct provision of services (both human services and
    physical services such as home remodeling)
Vouchers for the purchase of some services
Gifts or loans of equipment (e.g., hearing aids, prosthetic
    devices, wheelchairs)
Rebates on the purchase of some goods (e.g., automobiles)
    and services
Discounts on the purchase of certain services and goods
Tax exemptions or credits

Besides assistance through these programs, there are additional sub-categories. For example, in Japan rail transportation discounts are provided for persons with physical disabilities and bus discounts are available for persons with mental impairments.

Countries that provide benefits at the national level also provide benefits at other government levels, for example, state, province, county, or municipality. This produces an additional factor affecting the variation between countries in the assistance available for families with children with disabilities. Furthermore, beyond government-provided services, private groups receive public funds to provide certain services to some children and families. Additionally, in the absence of a universal health care system in a country, employment-based benefits provide certain forms of assistance, including health care and (to a considerably lesser extent) parental leave. This is true in the United States.

GENERAL ARRANGEMENTS

The financial assistance provided to children with disabilities and their families in each of the nine countries is described below in the context of the country's general social welfare system. In some countries, Sweden for example, the general welfare system is almost synonymous with the system for persons with disabilities. In other countries, while the general welfare system provides a framework, the assistance to persons with disabilities is quite separate. Given the relationship in each country between the general social welfare system and the programs for persons with disabilities, this chapter is longer than those following, first describing a country's general social welfare system and then turning to its services for persons with disabilities.

AUSTRALIA

In Australia social welfare programs were first provided by the federal government in 1908 under the Australian Constitution, which came into effect in 1901 and authorized legislation for what were called age and invalid pensions. In 1941, the Parliament provided a child endowment, a flat rate cash payment free of a means test, to parents for children after the first born. Federal unemployment and sickness benefits were provided in 1945. As in other industrialized countries, following the Second World War the range of benefits, allowances, and pensions grew at an increasing rate.

The first major involvement of the federal government as a direct service deliverer in the rehabilitation field was as a provider of vocational rehabilitation services in 1948. In the following decades, a variety of special laws were enacted, including the Disabled Persons Accommodation Act, 1963; Sheltered Employment Assistance Act, 1967; Handicapped Children Assistance Act, 1970; Handicapped Child Allowance, 1973; Handicapped Persons Assistance Act, 1974; Disability Services Act, 1986; and the Child Disability Allowance, 1987. The federal government is currently involved in a broad range of welfare programs designed to assist children, homeless people, older persons, people in crisis, and persons with disabilities. These programs, in general, either involve joint funding and administration with state and territory governments or the provision of grants and subsidies to local governments and non-government bodies.

Additionally, the state and territory governments and private welfare programs provide a range of welfare services, in many instances directed to the same population groups as those targeted by the federal government. The federal programs tend to supplement existing state efforts; however, in some instances the reverse is the case. Also, private welfare programs, some with government support, provide a range of services.

Three major federal government departments have responsibility for issues and programs related to persons with disabilities. The first is the Department of Community Services and Health, which funds state and local governments, rehabilitation programs, hearing services, health protection programs, and non-government service provision. The second is the Department of Employment, Education and Training, which provides labor market services, education funding to the states and territories, and supports non-government schools. The third is the Department of Social Security, which provides income security-related cash benefits and allowances. Third, the federal government established the Office of Disability, in 1966, which functions across the entire range of governmental activities through the Minister for Community Services and Health. This government-wide office is unique among the nine countries.

The Disability Services Act of 1986 was authorized to ensure that persons with disabilities receive the services necessary for them to achieve their maximum potential as members of the community and to be integrated into the community. The act is designed to achieve positive outcomes, such as increased independence, employment opportunities, and integration in the community; to promote a positive image of persons with disabilities and enhance their self-esteem; and to encourage innovation in the provision of services for persons with disabilities. Given the far-reaching goals of this act, it is being phased in over a 5-year period, 1987–1992.

The act authorizes both the provision of funding to the non-government and local government sectors and rehabilitation services though the federal government. For the purposes of funding the non-government sector, the act targets persons whose disabilities are attributable to an intellectual, psychiatric, sensory, or other physical impairment, or a combination of such impairments; are or are likely to be permanent; and result in substantially reduced capacity for communication or learning or mobility, and result in the need for ongoing services. For federal rehabilitation services, the target groups are persons between 14 and 65 years of age, who have disabilities that are attributable to an intellectual, psychiatric, sensory, or other physical impairment or combination of such impairments, and that result in substantially reduced capacity to obtain or retain unsupported paid employment or to live independently. Among the new services being provided under the act are accommodation support services, competitive employment training and placement services, independent living training services, information services, print disability services, recreation services, respite care services, supported employment services, and advocacy services.

In-home support services are provided in Australia under the Home and Community Care Act, 1985. While earlier legislation provided services primarily for older persons, the new act serves people of working age with a disability and families caring for children with disabilities. The act supports personal care, home care, home nursing, and transportation services, provided through local governments or non-government agencies.

States and territory governments all administer programs and services for people with disabilities and families who support a member with a disability. This is predominantly in the area of intellectual or developmental disability in both institutional and home-based settings. Under the Australian Constitution, education is a responsibility of the states. However, given its taxation authority, the federal government affects educational activities. Funds are provided to the states specifically for special education purposes. Funding is based upon the educational needs of children, including those with severe and profound disabilities, and provides for programs of integration and early special education. Generally, local governments are not providers of human services, although interest in service provision at this level is increasing, especially in provision of assistance to older persons.

Illustrative of a general trend in Australia's social welfare policy is the Child Disability Allowance introduced in 1987. Replacing an earlier means-tested program, the new allowance is universal, not taxed, and is provided for children with a range of disabilities. Parents or guardians who provide care at home for their children who require care and attention on a daily basis with an expectation that such services will be needed for a long period of time or permanently are eligible for this allowance. Parents may also receive the income-tested Family Allowance, Family Allowance Supplement, and a Health Care Card without affecting the Child Disability Allowance benefit.

CANADA

In Canada the federal constitution defines the powers and responsibilities of the federal and provincial governments in all areas, including those that relate to disability issues and programs. The general pattern is that the federal government shares the cost of specified services delivered by the provinces. These services and systems are designed by the province, often in the context of federal criteria for cost sharing. The provinces either implement services directly or indirectly through purchase of service agreements. In some provinces, local jurisdictions (municipalities, counties, regional governmental authorities) play a major role in both funding and delivery of social services, while in others their role is minimal.

The federal government: 1) delivers some global income security programs and unemployment insurance and related programs; 2) shares the cost of many health and social services with the provinces in ways that are defined by federal legislation and federal-provincial agreements; 3) supports research and development activities; 4) provides information and consultation services; and 5) is solely responsible for many programs involving veterans and Native people. Provincial governments: 1) have jurisdiction over hospitals, asylums, charities, and charitable institutions; 2) are responsible for elementary and secondary education; 3) provide direct services including institutions of all types, residential and special schools, financial assistance and welfare, community residential services, child welfare services, family support services, and adult protection services; and 4) fund and regulate provision of services by municipalities, and private for-profit and not-for-profit organizations.

Public elementary and secondary schools are operated by local authorities (both lay and religious) under provincial legislation. In many cases, community boards of various types oversee the operation of hospitals, residential and vocational services, child welfare programs, homes for older people, day-care centers, and so forth. The private for-profit sector is heavily involved in the delivery of human services.

The umbrella provided by the federal government leads to a human service system with many features that are consistent across the country. There are, however, considerable variations from province to province in terms of the range and types of specific services provided, rules of access to services, and the nature of the operators of the service.

The major funding and cost-sharing plans involving the federal and provincial governments include the Canada Assistance Plan, covering many health and social services, including home assistance, residential programs, child care, and child welfare services; the Federal-Provincial Fiscal Arrangements and Federal Post-Secondary Education and Health Contributions Act, covering many long-term adult residential care facilities, hospitals, and health insurance plans; and the Vocational Rehabilitation of Disabled Persons Act.

Provincial funding is brought to bear on service delivery in a number of ways including: 1) the direct delivery of social services by civil servants, particularly in institutions; 2) income maintenance programs; 3) child welfare and vocational rehabilitation services; 4) licensing and approval processes as a condition of funding, as well as licensing when no funding is involved; 5) cost-sharing with local governments and funding to private profit and not-for-profit organizations; and 6) purchase of service arrangements, focused upon individual service plans, and allocation of funds to families and individuals, either directly or through an intermediate agency. In general, provincial funding has been used for facilities, thus building a social service infrastructure that emphasizes congregate services and separation. There is an increasing tendency, however, toward the funding of "soft" services and for those services that are more community rather than institution focused.

Actual service delivery arrangements in Canada, while varying from jurisdiction to jurisdiction, generally involve: 1) provincially operated institutions, income maintenance, and child welfare services; 2) not-for-profit community agencies operating some forms of institutions and most residential services, sheltered workshops and community employment programs, family support, day care, and other nonmandatory programs; and 3) for-profit agencies and entrepreneurs involved in institutional services such as nursing homes and homes for special care.

Since the 1970s, there has been a definite trend away from such institutional services and toward community-based activities, particularly for persons with mental disabilities. For example, there have been major institutional closures in seven provinces, and scheduled closures in at least three more; in Newfoundland there are no children with mental disabilities in institutions, while in New Brunswick the single public institution for children has been closed. There is a shift to less restrictive and more enhancing environments for people who are seen as having the mildest disabilities. Such programs include supported independent living, work experience programs, job placement and supported employment, and integration into regular school classes. Through the building of support systems for families and individuals there is an increasing effort to bring all individuals with mental handicaps into the least restrictive and the most enhancing environment.

An increasingly important part of the framework of the national welfare systems is the Canadian Charter of Rights and Freedoms and the provincial human rights codes. Individually and together they define both individual entitlement and the nature of acceptable behavior of human services providers. The Charter guarantees people with disabilities equal protection and benefit of the law, freedom of movement and association, and protection from harm and cruel and unusual punishment. A number of the provincial human rights codes prohibit discrimination on the grounds of disability; most refer to physical disability, while some refer to both mental and physical disability.

Until the late 1980s, the major alternative for a family having financial difficulties in maintaining a child with disabilities at home was institutionalization. Support was provided to the institutions, not to the families. Increasingly, however, there are programs that provide support to the families. While such support is now becoming almost routine, there are extreme variations in the amount and type of assistance available. All Canadians have access to short- and long-term financial assistance and a public health insurance program. Among the types of assistance available in one or another province are: 1) monthly allowances paid to a family caring for a child with a severe impairment to assist with recurring extraordinary costs; 2) financial assistance for such special needs as specific equipment, assessment services, travel costs to services, and support workers; 3) financial assistance for special services and needs such as adaptive equipment and devices, assessment services, travel costs to special services, and hiring support workers to assist the individual; 4) subsidies in the payment of services that would otherwise be purchased by families at full price; and 5) tax exemptions and rebates for special items, motor vehicles, property taxes, income taxes (for those over the age of 21 and dependent), and deductions from income taxes for medical expenses and child care. A growing trend, although as yet a limited one, is the allocation of funds either directly to the family or on behalf of the family to a local agency.

ISRAEL

In Israel social services are provided by the central government agencies, which initiate the needed legislation, provide the budget, and oversee implementation. Actual service delivery is provided either directly by one of the central government agencies or delegated to municipal councils or private volunteer agencies.

The largest government ministry providing social services is the Ministry of Labor and Social Affairs, established in 1977, merging the activities of the Ministry of Labor, the Ministry of Social Welfare, and the National Insurance Institute. This unified ministry functions in three areas: 1) promoting the development and optimal utilization of the nation's human resources, 2) providing socio-economic development and advancement for individuals and groups, and 3) ensuring an effective system of social security. The Ministry is responsible for legislation and policy-making in these areas, supervising local services, and providing 75% of the budget for all services. These include services for older people, child care services, services for youth in distress, probation services for youth and adults, institutional care, and vocational and rehabilitation services for persons with physical or developmental disabilities.

The National Insurance Institute, although a part of the Ministry, is an independent, corporate body with its own property and funds. It provides old age and survivor's pensions, maternity benefits, work injury benefits, large families allowances, employees' children's allowances, unemployment insurance, disability insurance, child allowance and alimony payments, and general pensions. Insurance covers all Israeli residents, except housewives, from age 18 to pensionable age.

Health services are provided though the Ministry of Health and the National Workers Sick Fund, as well as by a number of smaller sick fund insurance agencies. Over 90% of the population is covered by the various health insurance programs. Heavy emphasis is placed upon preventive medical care through a network of over a thousand health clinics across the country.

Three principal laws form the framework for rehabilitation in Israel: the Compensation and Rehabilitation for Disabled Veterans Act of 1949, the Work Accident Act of 1954, and the General Disability Act of 1974. While the provisions of the first are administered through the Ministry of Defense, provisions of the other two are the responsibility of the National Insurance Institute. An additional distinction between programs for persons disabled as a result of military service and programs for all other persons with disabilities is the greater quantity and variety, as well as higher quality, of services for the veterans.

The Rehabilitation Services Administration of the Ministry of Labor and Social Welfare provides diagnostic assessment, vocational evaluation, personal and vocational adjustment services, training in activities of daily living, vocational training, job development and placement, and follow-up services. Rehabilitation Centers, Inc., is a government company that operates rehabilitation centers throughout the country and carries out projects with the Rehabilitation Services Administration, and public and private associations and organizations. An independent department provides services for persons with a mental handicap and supervises all public and private agencies providing services to this population. Similarly, a separate unit provides and supervises services for persons who are blind.

Some services are provided through non-government agencies. Additionally, agencies organized around a specific disability, usually by parents, provide for specific groups and their needs, for example those with neuromuscular handicaps, deafness, and blindness. Several years ago these organizations came together into a "roof" organization, a coalition of 22 parent groups, service agencies, and groups of persons with disabilities. Subsequently, they have split in two, one group consisting of groups of persons with disabilities and the other of parents' and service organizations.

Financial assistance to individuals with disabilities varies depending upon severity and type of disability, the individual's financial circumstance, and the previously noted matter of veteran status. In 1984, a law was enacted providing financial assistance for parents with a child between the ages of 3 and 18 who has a severe disability or a chronic illness; and, in 1988 the law was amended to include children from birth. The law is designed to encourage the family to raise the child at home. (The pension is not available to families whose child is institutionalized or in foster care.) For families whose child is in an institution, the Ministry of Labor and Social Services provides payments to allow them to visit the child on a regular basis.

Families of children with less severe impairments (as measured by limitations in activities of daily living) are only provided assistance through general programs for low-income families. Local governments and private agencies provide specific types of assistance, such as subsidies for the purchase of necessary adaptive equipment, necessary home repair, or alterations. Tax reductions are provided under various circumstances; given Israel's high tax rate, this can provide a substantial benefit to families. For example, parents of a child with severe mobility problems can purchase an automobile without paying the 200% tax.

JAPAN

In Japan the term "social welfare" appeared for the first time in the new constitution adopted after World War II. Article 25 of the Constitution states that "all people shall have the right to maintain minimum standards of wholesome and cultured living" and "The state shall make maximum effort to promote and expand social welfare, social security and public health services to cover every aspect of the life of the people." Six basic social welfare laws have been enacted to carry out this broad commitment: the Public Assistance Law or the Daily Life Security Law (1946 and 1950), the Child Welfare Law (1947), the Law for the Welfare of Physically Disabled Persons (1949), the Law for the Welfare of Mentally Retarded Persons (1963), the Law for the Welfare of Elderly Persons (1963), and the Law for Maternal and Child Welfare (1964). The Social Welfare Service Law of 1950 supplements these laws, delineating how they should be carried out.

Japan's health insurance system is broadly divided into three basic types of insurance programs. The Employees Health Insurance scheme covers all employees and dependents through one of three separate funds, to which employees and employers contribute. The National Health Insurance scheme is a form of government-sponsored contributory health insurance for persons who are not covered by any of the Employees' Insurance schemes. And, medical insurance for old persons is provided for under the 1983 Health Care Law for the Elderly.

Needs for income security are addressed by a public pension system, welfare allowances, and public assistance. In 1961, the National Pension scheme was established for self-employed persons and farmers, as well as others who had not been covered by any pension arrangements. Before then, public pensions had been only for employees. In addition, there are noncontributory social allowances to compensate for special needs, such as those of persons who have severe disabilities. The Public Assistance Law or Daily Living Security Law comes into play to provide a minimum income level as a supplement to the other available income security schemes. In addition, there are other public insurance systems, such as Unemployment Insurance and Workmen's Accident Compensation Insurance.

Social welfare services in Japan are provided through three levels of government: the Ministry of Health and Welfare as the central administrative body; the prefectural level; and at the level of the municipalities, towns, and villages. For activities that are viewed as requiring a certain standard of service, regardless of where the individual recipient lives, the major responsibility rests with the national government, with public agencies as the primary service providers. Voluntary agencies that have special status are allowed to run some of these services. Other services are not so strictly regulated by the government. Voluntary organizations, as well as local authorities, provide these services. Prior to 1985, the national government provided the bulk of the funding for the first level of services. In that year, costs were shifted to an even division between the national and the prefectural levels. The effort to increase the responsiveness of services to local needs was given as the rationale. However, some local officials have viewed this as primarily a load shifting device, complaining that little local discretion is allowed.

Prevention and early identification of disabilities are provided for under the Maternal and Child Health Law. These include prenatal care and testing for congenital disturbances in newborns. Universal mass-screening programs are conducted at several ages for the early identification of disabilities. These services are operated at the prefectural level with national government subsidies.

Early intervention services are provided under the Child Welfare Law. Generally, these services are community-based, with costs shared between the national and prefectural governments. Day-care services begin at age 3, with some local authorities providing programs for younger children.

Overall, the Ministry of Labor has responsibilities for assistance in employment. This had been limited to services for persons with physical disabilities. In the later 1980s, amendments to the Physically Disabled Persons Employment Promotion Law, now retitled Disabled Persons Employment Promotion Law, provide for coverage of persons with mental retardation. Among the provisions of the law are quota systems for the employment of persons with disabilities based upon the number of employees in a firm, and subsidies to employers for making necessary workplace modifications. The Employment Security Law and the Vocational Training Law provide for guidance and vocational training to registered physically disabled or mentally retarded individuals. Revisions, in the later 1980s, to the income security programs provide coverage for persons without any income because of a disability occurring before age 20.

The Ministry of Health and Welfare has overall responsibility for the administration of welfare services for persons with disabilities. Operation of the programs is through prefectural and municipal governments. Generally, local welfare offices serve a catchment area of 100,000 persons and provide services such as medical rehabilitation, technical aids, and placement in institutions or at community-based services. Services for persons with mental retardation are the responsibility of the Children and Families Bureau, which also has responsibility for all children, disabled and nondisabled, under 18 years of age. Services for persons with physical disabilities are the responsibility of a separate bureau.

Two types of financial assistance are provided at the national level to families with a child with a disability. These funds are means-tested and are available for families whose child with a disability lives with them. The first type of support is based upon the severity of the child's impairment, while the second is based upon the level of need for care and assistance. In addition to these national level sources of support, some local authorities provide benefits.

Tax deductions and subsidies are provided for families with a child with a disability. Sales tax exemptions, such as those for the purchase of an automobile, are allowed when the purchases are considered essential to the care of the child with a disability.

Medical expenses for children with physical disabilities are subsidized on a sliding scale by the Ministry of Health and Welfare. Medical expenses not covered by insurance schemes are supported by the government for persons with mental impairments.

Transportation costs on the national railways and domestic airlines are subsidized for persons with physical disabilities (and a necessary attendant), while public bus fares are subsidized for both those with physical impairments and mental retardation. Low-income families with a dependent who is disabled receive a discount on the Japanese Broadcasting Corporation broadcasting fee.

Subsidies are provided for certain daily living expenses, such as remodeling of bathrooms, purchase of electric wheelchairs and typewriters, tape recorders, and artificial limbs and other prostheses.

KENYA

As a nonindustrial country, Kenya does not have a national welfare system. There are unwritten cultural practices that differ from tribe to tribe. As discussed in Chapter 3, in general, persons with disabilities were seen as part of the tribal community and, thus, benefit from caring attitudes and practices. However, with the advent of a monetary economy, these practices have largely eroded.

The Ministry of Culture and Social Services provides some programs for people who are disadvantaged. For individuals and families with low incomes, as well as for persons with disabilities, the focus of these services is on promoting economic development and self-sufficiency. Thus, there are programs to encourage poultry raising, small retail businesses, and so forth. A similar focus on self-sufficiency characterizes the vocational rehabilitation program for persons with disabilities. A small program provides for emergency payments to individuals with disabilities and to their families. Each of these programs is funded and operated by the national government. Some local authorities have social welfare services, but for the most part these are limited.

The overall objectives of the vocational rehabilitation program are to help persons with disabilities in the necessary physical and psychological adjustments to society; to promote the practical participation of persons with disabilities in daily life by improving access to public buildings and transportation; to promote effective measures for prevention of disability and rehabilitation for persons with disabilities; and to promote national and international efforts to provide persons with disabilities necessary assistance, training, care, and guidance toward opportunities for work and participation in society. The program serves persons between the ages of 16 and 45, while those of school age are served through the Ministry of Education. Services include Industrial Rehabilitation Centres, Rural Vocational Rehabilitation Centres, and sheltered workshops.

Non-governmental organizations (NGOs) play a prominent role in social welfare services in general, as well as those specifically for persons with disabilities. Many of these, especially those that are church-sponsored, date to the colonial period. While many of them receive (limited) government financial support, outside funding and the availability of missionary personnel give the NGOs substantial advantages. Generally, services for persons with disabilities are categorically organized, for example, there are separate training facilities for persons with visual impairments, hearing impairments, and speech impairments. Small homes for persons with disabilities and regional boarding schools for youth with disabilities offer some measure of integration, as well as programs for persons who otherwise would remain unserved. While local governments do not provide services for persons with disabilities, they generally waive local taxes for any person with a disability who operates a business.

There is no general national system that provides assistance to meet the needs of children with disabilities or their families. The Division of Social Welfare of the Ministry of Culture and Social Services does provide some services to children identified as disadvantaged, including some children with disabilities. The children with disabilities include those with learning impairments, speech impairments, and sight impairments, as well as those with other physical impairments and mental handicaps. The Division provides both institutionalized and community-based services to these children in conjunction with the programs of various NGOs. Emergency assistance is provided on an occasional basis, although strong cultural and traditional family ties discourage seeking such assistance, even in the face of great necessity and the erosion of traditional forms of support.

A unique program in Kenya involves cooperation with the Danish Department of International Development Cooperation (DANIDA). The DANIDA/Kenya program, in effect since 1983, operates on the philosophy that the lives of persons with disabilities should be as close as possible to the lives of persons who do not have disabilities. To promote this principle, two organizational entities have been established: the Kenya Institute of Special Education and the Educational Assessment and Resource Services. The Institute, located outside of Nairobi, has programs that train special teachers and rehabilitation personnel to work with people with all types of disabilities, offer inservice courses to people working in all fields of disability, carry out research in special education and rehabilitation, maintain a roster of persons qualified to offer services to persons with disabilities, and set up laboratories to facilitate local production of special education materials and adaptive equipment. In the later 1980s, the Institute established a model farm, in recognition of the fact that some 80% of Kenyans live in rural areas and most earn at least a portion of their income from farming.

While the Institute has a single location serving the entire country, the Ministry of Culture and Social Services has a decentralized system of assessment and early intervention. In each province one of the assessment and early intervention centers serves as a nucleus and provides support for other Services programs in the province. One of the Services' activities is a network of "small homes" at which groups of students with disabilities live, near their school, returning to their parents' homes on the weekend.

SWEDEN

In Sweden the basic social welfare system is extensive and incorporates a concern for persons with disabilities. In presenting social welfare legislation concerning persons with disabilities, the government's perspective is that a handicap is not a characteristic of the person with the impairment. Rather, it is the relation between the impairment or injury and the environment of the person. This perspective—which moves the handicap from the individual to the environment—places the responsibility on both public and private entities to make their activities accessible. Thus, for the most part there are not special legislation, special services, or special organizations for persons with disabilities in Sweden. While national laws set entitlement, it is the municipalities that have the responsibility for the provision of services. For example, the Social Service Act states, "The municipality shall provide for those who due to physical or other reasons have profound difficulties in their daily living to participate in society and live like others. . . ."

The integration of services for persons with disabilities in the broad social welfare system is well illustrated in the programs for children with disabilities and their families. A tax exempt child allowance is paid for all children from birth until 16 years of age. In addition, a taxed child care allowance is paid to families of children under 16 years of age living at home who, because of their disability, require special supervision and care. The level of the allowance depends upon the extent of the care the child needs. Furthermore, all families with children can apply for a national-municipal housing allowance that is provided on the basis of family income, housing costs, number of children in the family, and other welfare benefits received. A home adjustment grant, not means-tested, is available to families with a child with a disability for the costs of home modifications.

The parental insurance scheme provides different forms of financial compensation to all parents when they stay at home to care for their child(ren). In general, this provides for 90% of the parents' earned income. (All benefits are paid to either the mother or father.) Benefits are available for parents to stay at home to care for children through their 4th birthday, and to care for a sick child through 12 years of age (16 if the child has a disability).

Public child care is provided for preschool-age (from birth to 6 years of age) children, and for afterschool activities (for children from 7 through 12 years of age). Children with special needs of support are given priority in such services. The goal is both to promote the integration of the children and to give family members extra support. Within such programs, children with disabilities may receive such special services as smaller groups, specially trained staff, personal assistance, adaptive equipment, transportation services, and so forth. Additionally, families with a child with a disability may apply for such social services as respite care, summer camps, home help services, and transportation services.

All Swedish citizens are covered by a national health insurance system, financed primarily through employer contributions. The goals of the system are to promote more equitable distribution of services, to finance them, and control them. In addition to the broad array of services available to the population in general through the social service organizations of the municipalities, special services are available to children with disabilities and their families through county habilitation teams. Such teams are organized to cut across various specialty organization lines—those based upon both category of disability and service function—as well as to provide a safety net for the children and their families.

Addressing the continuing question of the balance between regular services and the need for special services are the provisions of the Act on Special Services for Intellectually Handicapped Persons, enacted in the later 1980s. The act recognizes the needs for services for such individuals, provides additional assistance for them and their families, abolishes the use of group residential homes, and declares the expectation that persons with intellectual handicaps will live in homes integrated with the rest of the community. The act mandates that county councils provide five types of services for persons with intellectual handicaps, including advisory services, services at an activity center for those above school age who are not gainfully employed, respite care, foster care or boarding homes, and small group homes for adults identified as unable to live independently.

THE UNITED KINGDOM

In the United Kingdom the national government, acting through Parliament or statutory regulations, develops primary legislation that sets policies. The actual implementation of these policies falls largely to some 120 Local Authorities, which are run by locally elected members. Within the broad policy framework, each Local Authority has the authority to develop local practices to suit local needs.

Each Local Authority has a Local Education Authority that deals with all educational services for children and youth except for the universities, and has a Social Services Department that deals with a range of social and welfare services, including those for children and families, as well as people who are older, mentally ill, or physically or mentally handicapped. Local Social Security offices are centrally administered by the Department of Health and are not controlled by the local Social Service Departments. These offices administer the whole range of social security benefits and allowances, including unemployment benefits, attendance and mobility allowances, and a range of special payments for people with special needs, including persons with disabilities.

The National Health Service (NHS) is also independent of local authorities and is funded and administered by the Department of Health and Social Security via 14 Regional Health Authorities which include 220 Health Districts. The boundaries of the Health Districts do not necessarily correspond with those of the Local Authorities, nor do mechanisms of funding or processes of decision-making; thus, there is a need for cooperation and coordination between them. The NHS is currently going through a major review. While the outcome is uncertain, among the major proposals are those for more delegation of authority to the local level (e.g., from regional to district authorities and from district authorities to local hospitals); introduction of self-governing hospitals; reformed management arrangements and more rigorous audit practices; and the option for general practitioners to manage their own budgets. Children's services are not included as part of the "core" services all districts must provide. The result of the proposed changes may lead to increasing fragmentation of services for children, including those with disabilities, as well as a possible reduction in services considered too expensive and not cost-effective.

Local Housing Authorities come under the Department of the Environment via regional Housing Corporations. They provide most of the public sector housing. Since the 1980s, it has been the government policy to sell off these council accommodations to their own tenants, thus reducing the stock of public housing.

Employment services are not part of the local authorities and are administered directly by the Department of Employment through a range of specialist services. Recruitment and job finding is the responsibility of local Job Centres, organized into regional networks and a national network through the Training Commission.

In varying degrees, these different bodies incorporate services for persons with disabilities as part of their regular services. This is limited, however, due to differences in the operation of the various organizations, dissention between and within the various local bodies, inconsistencies between national government decisions and local implementation, and differences within the various organizations as to the extent that services for persons with disabilities should be regular services or be specialized. A further force of fragmentation is in the separation of services for persons with disabilities by diagnostic category. Toward addressing some of these issues of integration and coordination of services, the Labour Government in 1974 appointed a Minister with specific responsibility for persons with disabilities. In 1979, the new Conservative Government made this one of the responsibilities of the Minister for Social Security.

Until the later 1980s, the legislative base for services to persons with disabilities has largely resided in legislation designed for the public as a whole, with only sections or clauses of acts of Parliament specifically concerned with services for persons with disabilities. For example, this was true of the Education Act, the National Health Service Acts, and the Health and Public Services Acts. The first major act of Parliament specifically concerned with the needs of persons with disabilities was the 1970 Chronically Sick and Disabled Persons Act. The act placed a statutory obligation on Local Authorities to identify persons with disabilities in their area; to make an assessment of their needs; to meet these needs by means of physical adaptations to homes, such as ramps, widening of doors, or installation of downstairs bathrooms or telephones. In addition, the act, while not requiring specific funding, required new public buildings to be constructed with the access needs of persons with disabilities in mind. The extent to which the act has been implemented has varied greatly from area to area, despite efforts by the national government and disability organizations to remind local authorities of their responsibilities.

To meet the problem of uneven implementation, in 1986 the Disabled Persons Services, Consultation and Representation Act was passed. It requires a Local Authority to assess the needs of a person with disabilities and his or her caregiver(s) on request. The Local Authority must assess the individual's needs for help in the home, leisure activities, assistance with transportation, aids and assistance, and other day-to-day living requirements. This act marks the first provision for the needs of the individual with a disability and those of his or her caregiver(s) to be assessed separately. Furthermore, persons with disabilities can ask for a representative to be appointed on their behalf during the assessment process. A number of Local Authorities are working with voluntary organizations to recruit, train, and support these representatives.

As in many countries, the transition from comprehensive school-age services to adult services is problematic. The Disabled Persons Act does ensure that a Local Authority's Social Services Department is involved in the pre-school leaving assessment carried out by the Local Education Authority according to the provisions of the 1981 Education Act. While the Disabled Persons Act requires assessment, including assessment of the needs of persons transferring from long-term residential institutions to community services, it imposes no statutory obligation to provide the services identified by the assessment. The provisions of the act, however, provide for representation of persons with disabilities by an advocate of their own choosing. This provision is seen as a major step forward in helping youth who are transferring to adult services to negotiate their needs with the Local Authorities.

In the United Kingdom, families with a child with disabilities are entitled to certain special allowances from the Department of Health. These are not means-tested; eligibility depends upon the severity of the child's disability. Families that also have low incomes are eligible for additional support from the social security system.

The main disability allowances include the Attendance Care Allowance, the Mobility Allowance, the Invalid Care Allowance, and the Severe Disablement Allowance. The Attendance Care Allowance is tax free and is paid at two rates—one is a day or night rate, the other is a day and night rate. It is provided for children over 2 years of age (or for adults) who have extra care needs over and above what would be usual for a person of the particular age group. The allowance can be paid on a part-time basis, for example when a child living at a residential school is home during a holiday period.

The Mobility Allowance is a tax free weekly payment available to persons with disabilities between 5 and 75 years of age. Eligibility depends upon inability to walk and the allowance is paid both to persons living in hospitals or in residential care. Some families use their allowance to lease or help purchase a car.

The Invalid Care Allowance is paid to family members who are unable to work because of the responsibility of caring for a person with severe disabilities.

The Severe Disablement Allowance is paid to people who cannot work because of long-term illness or disability and who cannot claim sickness or disability benefits because they have not paid sufficient insurance contributions. To be eligible for this allowance, persons must be 80% disabled; in practice, this usually means that the persons eligible for this allowance receive Attendance or Mobility Allowance benefits. While this is an adult allowance, young people over the age of 16 can receive it if they are still in school or college. Persons can receive this allowance as "therapeutic earnings," while working up to 15 hours a week.

Parents of children with disabilities who are under 16 years of age may receive special help from the Family Fund. This independent trust administers funds on behalf of the government, providing payments for special needs such as holidays, driving lessons, home adaptations, and special equipment.

The Social Security Act was implemented in 1986. Intended to rationalize a complex and out-of-date social security system, disability organizations are concerned that it may leave many persons with disabilities worse off than previously. Among its provisions are general income support for families who do not have enough money to live on; family credit for working people, designed to boost their income; the Social Fund, which provides exceptional needs payments, including regular support, crisis loans, and community care grants; and the housing benefit, which helps low-income families pay for their rent and local taxes. In addition, the Independent Living Fund, administered by the Disablement Income Group together with the Department of Health and Social Services, makes payments for personal and domestic help needed by persons with severe disabilities to remain at home.

The special needs of families with a child with a disability are highlighted in one of a series of 1989 reports by the Office of Population and Census Surveys on the lives of persons with disabilities in the United Kingdom. The report found that parents of children with disabilities were less likely to work and, if they were employed, were likely to earn less than other parents. Three-quarters of the single parents in the survey relied solely upon state benefits for their family income. Furthermore, the majority of families incurred additional expenses because of the presence of a child with a disability. Generally, these extra expenditures went for travel, food, laundry, and fuel, with the latter two needs creating the major expenses. Disability organizations in the UK see the report's findings as strengthening the argument for a national disability income program.

THE UNITED STATES OF AMERICA

In the United States of America federal legislation—much of it initially enacted through the New Deal's Social Security Act of 1935—sets the framework and provides a portion of the funding for basic social welfare programs. The current Aid to Families with Dependent Children (AFDC) program, established by the Social Security Act of 1935 as Aid to Dependent Children (ADC), provides cash relief to families with little or no income. The name was changed to AFDC in 1950 when a caretaker grant was added. Since 1961, states have had the option of providing aid to families with an unemployed father in the home; to date just over half the states have taken this option. AFDC is administered by the states under federal guidelines, with funding from both federal and state resources. States are allowed wide latitude in setting both benefit levels and eligibility requirements, which creates a wide disparity among the states.

Medicaid is also authorized under the Social Security Act (Title XIX). It is designed to meet the medical needs of persons receiving public assistance by paying for needed medical services or equipment. All recipients of AFDC are eligible to receive Medicaid, as are certain persons with disabilities. Additionally, slightly more than half of the states provide assistance to persons with other medical needs. The Medicaid program is funded through both federal and state resources.

Medicare, also authorized under the Social Security Act (Title XVIII), is the largest health care program in the United States. It provides health insurance to workers with disabilities and to retired workers over the age of 65 and to dependents of these recipients. This program is funded through a payroll tax on employees and employers and by some recipient (co)payments.

Food stamps provide assistance to low-income families through a monthly allotment of coupons that can be redeemed for various food and some household products. Most persons with incomes below 130% of the poverty line qualify. The program is administered by the states with funding for the basic cost provided by the federal government and the states providing administrative funds.

The Supplemental Food Program for Women, Infants, and Children (WIC) is administered by the states with combined federal and state funding. This program is designed to prevent disabilities through the promotion of better nutrition among low-income pregnant women and their babies.

The current framework of services for persons with disabilities stems largely from federal laws passed in the 1970s, many grafted onto earlier legislation. The laws reflect an emerging national consensus that persons with disabilities should receive needed services within their local communities. For example, the Rehabilitation Act of 1973 (PL 93-112) is commonly referred to as the civil rights law for persons with disabilities. In several sections it prohibits discrimination against persons of all ages with disabilities on the part of programs receiving various forms of federal financial assistance. In 1990, pending before the Congress is the Americans with Disabilities Act (ADA) that will extend the protections to private employment, places of public accommodation, and housing.

The two major federal income maintenance programs benefitting individuals with disabilities are the Supplemental Security Income (SSI) and Social Security Insurance for Adult Disabled Children (SSDI) programs. SSDI, established in 1956, provides payments to children with disabilities, 18 years of age and older, of retired, disabled, or deceased workers. Children under 18 are eligible for payments under the Social Security Disability Program provided that a parent who is retired, disabled, or deceased participated in the Social Security taxation program.

SSI was established in 1972 under the Social Security Act (Title XVI). It establishes a base federal income support level for persons who are blind, disabled, or older. Eligibility is limited to persons who acquire a disability before age 22 and who are not capable of "substantial gainful employment." Children with disabilities are also eligible for benefits under SSI, but this is largely a means-tested allotment based on parental income. Thus, only children of very-low-income families qualify.

Persons with disabilities can qualify for financial support through the Supplemental Security Income (SSI) program. This program can help offset the family's living and care-related expenses. A number of states make cash assistance available to caregiving families. And family members may also benefit financially from certain worker benefits plans established by employers.

The major health care program for persons with disabilities is funded through Medicaid. Additional services are provided through block grants to states through the Maternal and Child Health Care program. In most states an individual is automatically eligible for Medicaid if she or he receives SSI. In the other states, most adults with developmental disabilities or mental retardation are eligible for Medicaid.

Regarding health benefits, children with developmental disabilities or chronic illnesses face a more complex situation in that family income is taken into account for eligibility if the child lives at home. A 1982 amendment to the law governing the Medicaid program allows states to provide support for home care of children who would otherwise be served in an institutional setting at an equal or higher cost; a dozen states have opted into this arrangement. (In most cases, these states have narrowly defined eligibility for this program.) A substantial portion of health care benefits for the entire population is provided through employee health care programs. While in the past many of these programs excluded or limited the options for children with a disability, currently this is less often the case.

The Developmental Disabilities Act of 1970 and subsequent amendments provide an array of services for persons with developmental disabilities. At the federal level, developmental disabilities are defined as severe disabilities manifested prior to age 22 that result in substantial functional limitations in major life areas and that engender the need for extended or lifelong services. Grants are made to the states to provide services such as case management, community living, and advocacy. Amendments in 1984 focused on helping persons with developmental disabilities achieve maximum independence, productivity and integration into the community, including employment-related activities.

The Social Security Amendments of 1971 authorized services in institutional settings (Intermediate Care Facilities) to be paid by Medicaid, thus shifting the major part of the financial burden from the states to the federal government. Since then, the federal government has made it possible for states to shift these resources from large separate facilities to small community-based settings. While numerous institutions still exist, states are increasingly opting to develop community-centered responses to the needs of persons with disabilities, including highly supportive arrangements for those with severe disabilities.

The Vocational Rehabilitation Act, which dates to the early 1920s (most recently PL 98-221, 1986), provides for vocational rehabilitation of persons disabled in industry to assist in their return to employment. With various amendments, this program provides an array of federally supported and state operated programs for assessment, counseling, job placement, follow-up, sheltered workshops, and supported employment.

These federally based programs are also complemented by programs instituted and funded at the state level. For example, most of the states fund one or another form of family support programs. These programs vary greatly as to eligibility, type and level of benefits, and number of persons covered. While most offer only a restricted set of services, about 20 states make financial assistance available to families to offset care-related expenses. Of these 20, some offer this type of assistance as a periodic cash grant, while others utilize voucher systems. Some states combine cash assistance and voucher payments with support services. Typically, states that offer financial assistance also provide a range of other support services. Even so, the level of support varies greatly, as does the number of families covered.

In the private sector, increasingly available cafeteria plans for employee benefits allow workers to opt for a mix of benefits that sometimes include family support services. Overall, although states are improving their response to family needs, the resources invested in family supports are far less than what is spent on "out-of-home" alternatives.

URUGUAY

In Uruguay Article 40 of the Constitution states, "The family is the basis of our society. The State shall ensure that its moral and material stability is kept, towards a better formation of children within Society." It is within this framework of the centrality of the family that an array of social welfare programs are established, including the General Retirement Pension System, which provides for pensions for both persons over 70 years of age and those whose disabilities affect their ability to work; the Children's Code, which provides a variety of child protection services; and various allowance programs, including family and maternity benefits, allowances for spouses of public servants, and allowances for persons who have had industrial accidents. The Social Security System is administered through the Ministry of Labor and Social Security, which is responsible for policy-making, and by local agencies, public and private. The principles of the social security system are solidarity—that is, inclusion of all residents; universality—that is, equal coverage for all individuals; and sufficiency—that is, providing levels of support commensurate with individual need. The system is established under Article 195 of the Constitution, and operates through the Banco de Prevision Social (Social Security Bank). The Bank provides old age benefits, survivors' benefits, certain forms of disability benefits, retirement pensions and allowances, maternity benefits, children's allowances, and family benefits including a marriage premium and spouse allowance. The family allowance is paid from the time pregnancy is verified through the child's 18th year. Families with a child with mental retardation or some other forms of disability are entitled to twice the regular allowance, for the life of the child. While the conception of the various programs is quite broad, the actual resources provided are limited. For families with a child with a disability, these limited national programs are supplemented by some local government programs as well as by various private programs.

CONCLUSION

As indicated in the introduction to this chapter and illustrated by the review of social welfare provisions in the nine countries, there is great variety among provisions in terms of: 1) the extent to which programs for persons with disabilities are integral with the general social welfare schemes or stand apart from them; 2) the extent, type, and variety of such programs; 3) the structures and forms of service delivery; and 4) the philosophy that undergirds the programs. At the most general level, there seem to be some common tendencies across the nine countries. These include: 1) a trend toward access to common or general services, 2) growing fiscal constraints amidst expansion of service programs, 3) increased development of community-based program designs, and 4) a growing recognition of the need to support the family with a child with a disability. And, of course, often there is a substantial gap between the provisions of legislation and program design and the realities of services for families and children.

REFERENCES

Duncan, B., & Woods, D. (1987). *Social security disability programs: an international perspective* (Austria, Canada, Finland, Israel, Sweden, The Netherlands, Federal Republic of Germany, England). Monograph 41. New York: Rehabilitation International and International Exchange of Experts and Information in Rehabilitation, World Rehabilitation Fund, Inc.

5

Informing Families

This chapter surveys the formal systems that provide families with information about disability-related issues. As the Conference representatives from Canada point out, however, the most pervasive source of information about disability to families is neither a service nor a support. Rather, it is an integral part of each culture's patterns and biases, the understandings and misunderstandings in everyday life, portrayed in the media, expressed in professional advice, and so forth. This cultural pattern provides the basic information—or at least the framework within which particular information is provided—to parents of a child who has a disability.

In each of the nine countries, the formal systems that provide information about disability exist primarily through the systems of prenatal care and general hospitals. Overall, where these are extensive and well-developed, considerable information is available to parents regarding their child's particular condition. Where this is less the case, the number of parents provided with such information are fewer. Beyond this general observation, countries differ in the nature of the information provided and its sources.

AUSTRALIA

In Australia there is no formal centralized system that provides families with specific information about the disability of their child. Provision of information generally occurs at state and local levels. A number of non-government sector groups, including parent-run groups, provide information; some are funded by the federal and some by state governments. The federal government also funds such national agencies as the Disabled Peoples' International, the Australian Council for Rehabilitation of the Disabled, and the National Association for People with Intellectual Disabilities, which function as coordinating organizations with local affiliates in the various states. The local agencies generally play the most active role in direct contact with families. In addition, some state governments have coordination units or advisory bodies that can also refer individuals to agencies that provide information.

Local family doctors, however, continue to be the primary source of professional advice. General practitioners usually refer families to specialist pediatricians or to metropolitan children's hospitals for diagnosis. In those states where developmental disabilities services have been regionalized, specialist teams are often found. They usually have developed close links with local or regional hospitals and thus, may be called upon as soon as a child is diagnosed as having a developmental disability or to provide a diagnosis. These services may also include the provision of programs, support, and information for families. If a child is thought to have a specific disability, such as autism or cerebral palsy, referrals may be made to a non-governmental agency that provides services to people with the identified disability. In Victoria, New South Wales and some other states, ethno-specific agencies provide outreach information services and advocacy to families. These agencies link families to other services and facilitate a better understanding of the needs of families from non-English speaking backgrounds. Additionally, parent groups for different language groups create an informal network of support.

CANADA

In Canada most families receive formal information about their child's disability from health and education professionals in the context of major events and stress, that is, prenatal diagnosis, at birth, or in the early years of school. For the most part, this information is profoundly colored by negative interpretations of disability and frequently relates to life and death issues for the child. In a few communities, groups such as Parents-to-Parents, an organization of parents of children with disabilities, provide advice and information.

The most extensive information about disability comes from the G. Allan Roeher Institute of the Canadian Association for Community Living. A private organization with affiliates throughout Canada, some of the association's work in this area is supported by the federal government. This includes a series of monographs that deal extensively with overcoming the handicapping nature of the environment and ways to prevent societal responses from causing or aggravating handicap. In addition, parent and professional groups that are concerned with specific disabilities also produce a wide array of information and attempt to stay in communication with parents.

A variety of associations and groups are involved in developing and disseminating information. In some professional service agencies, both those with a specific disability focus and those more generally concerned with child welfare, staff with various titles (e.g., Family Support Worker, Special Needs Worker, Case Coordinator) provide information to parents. Issue-oriented groups (e.g., the Integration Action Group, Concerned Friends of Ontario Citizens in Care Facilities) provide information and support to individuals and parents regarding gaining access to the community. Other groups (e.g., Pilot Parents and Parents-to-Parents) provide information to parents from the earliest days of identification of the child's disability. Early provision of information, the use of parent groups, and emphasis upon both the potential of the child with a disability and the handicapping consequence of society's negative responses are growing trends in Canada.

ISRAEL

In Israel the early identification of disability is an important basic step in the provision of services to families. Various service providers might be involved in the process depending upon the nature of the impairment. If the impairment is detected during pregnancy or soon after birth, the pediatric or neonatal units in the hospitals usually provide the initial primary information to the parents. These units are responsible for referring the parents and child to the appropriate child developmental clinic in their community or geographic area and for connecting them with one of the mother and child centers that exist throughout Israel.

The mother and child centers serve all mothers and children in their area, are free to all, and have primary prevention and early diagnosis among their major responsibilities. They also provide free care to pregnant women. In cases where the impairment is identified later in the child's life, the referral may be initiated by the public health nurse at one of the mother and child centers. On the basis of such screening, referral would be made to a specialized child developmental clinic.

There are 18 child developmental clinics dispersed throughout Israel, sponsored by different government and public institutions. While the range of services may vary from one clinic to the other, all have a common goal of evaluation, diagnosis, and follow-up of children with developmental problems under the age of 5. After a diagnosis, either the required direct services for the child are provided by that center or a referral is made to a center with the needed specialty.

Information is also provided by parent groups affiliated with specific disability groups and other voluntary organizations. Organizations that serve children with specific disabilities include AKIM (mental disabilities), ILAN (neuromuscular disabilities), NITZAN (learning disabilities), and SHEMA (hearing impairments). While national in scope, these organizations operate through local groups, primarily consisting of parents supported by social work professionals. For example, AKIM has 32 branches.

Several government groups provide information about disabilities to parents. Among them, the National Insurance Institute provides printed brochures explaining the various laws and rights offered to different client populations. While Arab families receive the same information, there is no written material in Arabic.

JAPAN

In Japan once pregnancy is confirmed a maternal and child handbook is given to the expectant mother by the Health Department of the local government. All the health information concerning the mother during pregnancy and about the child during preschool years is recorded in this handbook. All expectant mothers and their newborns are entitled to free periodic health check-ups. Mass child screenings are done by the Health Department at 3 or 4 months of age, at 1½ years, and at 3 years of age to detect disabilities or risk factors in children so that early intervention services may be provided. Though in its initial stages, this health system is designed to ensure continuous and systematic follow-up. The system is set up to work so that a preschool-age child with an identified impairment will be referred to a special day care facility for preschool children with disabilities.

To improve the effectiveness of the information system, in the late 1970s the Ministry of Health and Welfare began to subsidize local authorities in the establishment of multidisciplinary diagnostic, treatment, and consultation centers. Such centers have outpatient clinics staffed by various professionals and day care centers for youth with mental retardation and physical disabilities. Social workers at the centers coordinate interagency activities and provide consultation services to other agencies. At the centers, parents can obtain information and advice concerning child rearing, financial assistance, and assistance in gaining access to various services. The center's public health nurse often arranges informal parent support groups. These groups provide a source of information and support to parents newly involved with a child with a disability.

KENYA

Information dissemination is a major problem in Kenya as in most nonindustrial countries. This is a matter of limited resources, information systems, and grassroots personnel to disseminate information. Organized support services for specific disabilities do not exist. And the attitudes of some ethnic groups toward disability make it difficult for families to discuss problems openly. Most families, therefore, do not seek or share information. Beyond this attitudinal issue, many families do not know where and how to seek information.

In a positive direction, the Ministry of Education has established assessment centers in many districts to which all children with disabilities can come. It is projected that by the early 1990s, about two-thirds of parents with children with a disability will be served by or have access to these centers.

An important resource is the Voice of Kenya, the national broadcasting service. It has broadcast programs about disability on both radio and television. However, the limited availability of radios or television sets circumscribes the reach of these efforts. In Nairobi, the Civitan Foundation has begun to provide some information services to parents.

SWEDEN

In Sweden the social welfare office in the community and the Board of Provisions and Services for the Disabled of the County Council provide information to parents of children with disabilities. The focus of information concerning disability is to encourage the family to raise the child at home. Information about disability is also given by other formal care providers. Parent associations have an important role in this area. They organize seminars and conferences, publish pamphlets and monographs, and make videotapes about various disabilities.

The local government unit (e.g., the County Council in Stockholm) is responsible for the provision of information to families. Courses are provided to parents, and close collaboration is set up between the parent education team of the council and parent associations. Special efforts are made to ensure that information is culturally relevant to the family. For example, an "immigrant secretary" supported by a committee of specialists functioning as a consultant team works with families with a child with a disability. The committee provides information about services offered through the County Council in the five major immigrant languages. In an effort to reach out to immigrant families, the law that regulates general government administration affords every non-Swedish speaking immigrant the right to have an interpreter for any dealings with an official service or authority at government expense. Also, parent education courses have been developed for immigrant parents in some districts to provide information about services. One of the outcomes of these courses has been to increase the sensitivity of agency staff to the needs of the various immigrant communities.

UNITED KINGDOM

In the United Kingdom the Education Act of 1981 introduced important principles of access to information on the assessment of children with special education needs. For the first time, parents in the UK had the right to see the professionally developed Statement of Educational Needs (the outcome of the formal assessment provided for under the act) and to contribute their views to the statement on an equal basis with professionals. While far-reaching in terms of rights, the provision of information to parents and their participation in decision-making have yet to be fully realized. A number of local authorities have projects underway to increase the effectiveness of these rights. These projects include the use of trained volunteers as counselors or advisers to parents, and the restructuring of both the way in which the information is provided and the format used. As a result of available information, in some areas of the country increased parental involvement in agency planning and evaluation has taken place.

Information about disability from health and social services agencies is increasingly being made available to parents. In the health area, parental access to information continues to be limited by the National Health Services Act of 1977 provision that personal health records are technically the property of the Secretary of State. In reality, however, their availability varies according to the practice of individual health care providers. In the social services field, the Data Protection Act of 1966 has radically changed access to social services records. Parents now have access to social services records and information, and a later ruling by the Minister for Health confirms that this right covers access to the records of persons with mental handicaps.

THE UNITED STATES OF AMERICA

In the United States of America as in the United Kingdom, the basic legislation for the provision of educational services for children with handicapping conditions incorporates the requirement of a planning document (the Individualized Education Program [IEP]), which is meant to itemize the student's needs, the service response, and the expected outcomes. Parents have both input into the preparation of this plan and involvement in its implementation. With the 1986 Education of the Handicapped Act Amendments (PL 99-457), which extended earlier legislation, children with disabilities are provided for from birth, and information is available to the parents of all children with disabilities. As these provisions are only now being implemented, it is not clear as yet whether they will be comprehensive or restricted to educational activities.

Unlike in Israel, there is no national system of maternal and child health care in the United States. Programs therefore vary among individual states and within states among communities. Many hospitals and some governments at the local level have prenatal programs and early identification activities. A few hospitals have developed peer assistance systems where a parent who has given birth to a baby with a particular disability is offered the opportunity to meet with other parents with an older child with a similar disability. Many of the disability-specific organizations have similar outreach efforts including periodic meetings and newsletters. Both the hospital programs and those of these organizations have had limited success in reaching parents who have low incomes or who are people of color.

In recognition of the needs of families for information related to disability, the Education of the Handicapped Act was amended in 1983 to establish a national network of Parent Training and Information (PTI) Programs. This system was envisioned as a parent-to-parent peer network that would provide information and training to parents so that they could participate more effectively with professionals in meeting the educational needs of their children. At present, there are PTI centers in most states. These regional centers and a national back-up center provide training, technical assistance, and development of materials.

The 1983 Amendments also authorized the establishment of a National Information Center for Handicapped Children and Youth (NICHCY). This center provides free information for parents, educators, advocates, and other caregivers. The center both publishes materials, including directories of statewide services, and responds to individual questions.

URUGUAY

In Uruguay at the national level, the National Commission on Habilitation and Rehabilitation, conducted under the leadership of the Ministry of Public Health, develops national policy, collects pertinent material, and disseminates some information. Local hospitals, particularly those in the urban centers, are a source of information to parents. Since 1981, the provision of educational services to children with handicapping conditions has incorporated a required parental involvement component. Additionally, the various special education schools provide information both to the parents of the children attending their school and to the public at large through publications and meetings.

Private organizations play an important part in the development and dissemination of information. In all organizations the strengthening of the family as the central unit of support for the child with a disability underlies the activities. Among these organizations, major work has been conducted by the Inter-American Childrens' Institute, the PATH (Partners in Appropriate Technology for the Handicapped) Centers, the National Association for the Mentally Retarded Child, the National Federation of Associations of Disabled Persons, and the Center for the Integration of Disabled Persons. These organizations, closely intertwined in initiation and operation of projects, involve in differing degrees a mix of professionals and parents.

CONCLUSION

In each of the countries, local private organizations provide information to families. The extent to which governmental bodies do so varies among the nine countries, as does the type of agency—health, social services, educational. Only to a limited extent in any of the countries is the information provided sensitive to the needs of differing cultural groups.

6

Education

In each of the nine countries, there is a universal system of publicly supported education within which educational services for children with handicaps is provided. Both the overall systems and the services for students with handicapping conditions vary as to the ages of children served and the level of government that is responsible.

AUSTRALIA

In Australia the Constitution mandates that education is a direct responsibility of the states. Because the federal government controls income tax collection, the major source of government revenue, it is able to have an influence on state policies through the provisions governing the disbursement of these funds. Among these are specific provisions for funding to the states for special education purposes. This includes funding for: the special needs of children with severe and profound disabilities, early childhood programs for students with disabilities, and the integration of special education into regular education programs. The federal government also funds non-government schools.

137

Early intervention, therapy, and educational services for the most part are provided through the state governments. In many states, these services are part of the activities of the regional diagnosis and outreach centers. Additionally, some states fund non-government organizations to provide early education or intervention. The model of early education service differs within each state and between states. In some instances, the services are center-based and parents bring their children to the center. In others, there are home-based services through visiting teachers and therapists.

Once a child reaches school age (which varies from state to state), the separate special education system in all states provides special education through special schools. There is a growing move toward the integration of students with disabilities into regular education programs. Since 1984, in Victoria, children with disabilities have had the right to be educated in regular schools. Both Victoria and New South Wales, in particular, have allocated additional funds to provide support for integration, including integration aides who work in regular classrooms.

CANADA

In Canada there are clear distinctions between public education and early childhood services in terms of policy, funding, and operations. A major difference is that publicly supported education is a universal, mandatory system, while early intervention, early childhood education, and other services which are defined, generally, as "special services," are neither mandatory nor universally available or funded.

Early intervention and therapy services oriented toward developing a child's skills or capabilities are provided through social services and health agencies. By and large, funding for such services is from provincial government departments with cost sharing arrangements with the federal government. The services are provided by a wide diversity of providers, varying considerably from jurisdiction to jurisdiction—provincial government departments or institutions, municipal agencies, nonprofit and for-profit agencies, public hospitals, and health agencies.

During the 1980s there have been dramatic changes in the nature of community intervention services. While by and large the community and educational systems are still characterized by segregated services that emphasize special and therapeutic interventions by professionals, in more and more communities change is significant. In a growing number of jurisdictions, agency-based interventions and therapeutic services are being replaced or supplemented by itinerant services at the home, with an emphasis on developing the "teaching" skills of the family.

Information and instruction are brought to the family and others who are involved in the child's life. There are increasing numbers of professionals and paraprofessionals who come to the home, develop teaching strategies with the family, provide instruction in implementing these strategies, and help interpret information from other professionals so that families can make sense of it. At its best, this type of support combines excellent professional services with the power of natural environments and the family. The emphasis then shifts from isolated teaching and therapy to surrounding the child with people who teach and instruct in the natural course of events. Rather than programs, the events and occasions of everyday life become the contexts for teaching. For example, meals are occasions for families to spend time together eating, rather than being feeding programs.

Early childhood education (nursery and day care) services are defined across the country as community and social services. In some provinces, the provincial government not only licenses operations, but funds some to ensure that families with low incomes have access. In others, the provincial government's role is restricted to licensing.

With considerable variations from community to community, day-care and nursery services are operated by nonprofit and for-profit agencies and by municipalities. Where programs are available at all, they may be full-day or half-day, open to infants or restricted to toddlers, and offered in centers and/or home-based settings. Many communities have no formal early childhood education programs.

Historically, and frequently today, day-care and nursery programs have not been available to children with special needs. Where they have been available, they have been congregated, segregated programs operated either by institutions, therapeutic/rehabilitation centers, or parent associations. Increasingly, this is changing.

A number of parent associations are dismantling or changing their segregated centres—welcoming nonhandicapped children into their programs or working with regular centers to assist them in welcoming children with special needs. In addition, early intervention and therapeutic services are offering advice and assistance to regular centers and programs. In some areas, provincial funding is increased when regular centers have spaces for children with special needs.

These changes can have dramatic consequence for children and families. Early childhood programs become more accessible, generally and geographically, to families. Children with special needs and nonhandicapped children spend considerable and intimate time together—they grow together rather than apart. A growing number of early childhood educators are making the case to educational authorities that a child with special needs should learn and grow up with nonhandicapped peers.

Public elementary and secondary schools are operated by local authorities (school boards) under provincial legislation. With some variations, two types of school boards serve communities—public and separate (Roman Catholic). School funding comes from federal, provincial, and local taxation. Some jurisdictions provide programs beginning with kindergarten. The age for mandatory school attendance (and leaving school) varies across jurisdictions. The language of instruction in classes, used in general in the schools, and used by school boards varies locally and from province to province. In addition to English and French, there is growing recognition of aboriginal languages and those of other major cultural groups.

Until the 1980s, many schools for young people with special needs were operated by parent associations. Gradually, these schools have been integrated into provincial legislation governing all schools, and the students are educated under the authority of local school boards. For some young people who live in residential and institutional settings, schooling is provided in those settings, sometimes by local school authorities. Separate provincially operated schools continue for some students with special needs, particularly those with visual and/or hearing impairments.

For Canadians with developmental disabilities, for the most part the education system is now integrated at the systems level, that is, the education of students with disabilities is the responsibility of the local education authority. Integration at the systems level is not complete, however. For instance, in metropolitan Toronto, special schools for students with developmental disabilities are operated by a metropolitan-level school authority, rather than by the local school boards that operate elementary and secondary schools.

Integration into the regular school is less advanced, however, though advances have been considerable in specific areas across the country. In Newfoundland and Labrador, for example, there have been no separate special schools for children with developmental disabilities since the early 1980s. Across the country, however, special schools operated by public school systems are quite common. Gradually, different classifications of students have been moved from special schools to special classes in regular schools. Integration at the school level varies from province to province, within each province, and between school boards, public and separate, serving the same geographic area.

Integration at the classroom level is becoming the placement of choice of increasing numbers of parents, although it is far from universal or even common. This change in demand has been actively encouraged and aided by the Integration Action Group (a network of local parent/professional coalitions); the local, provincial, and national Associations for Community Living; and the Centre for Integrated Education and Community.

In response, and on occasion in anticipation, local and provincial education authorities are making severe to profound changes. At the provincial level, New Brunswick has been a leader. In some local school boards across the country, integration into the regular classroom is the assumed mode of change, rather than the result of protracted confrontations between families and authorities. Exemplary school board approaches exist across the country. Among the better known are the Woodstock district in New Brunswick, and several Roman Catholic separate school boards in southern Ontario (Hamilton-Went-worth, Waterloo County, and Wellington County). (For a discussion of some of these activities see Stainback, Stainback, & Forest, 1989.) Other efforts are underway in British Columbia and Saskatchewan.

The development of community and professional expertise in the inclusion movement has been fostered by interactions among the many individual and organizational leaders within parent and professional organizations. This expertise has been furthered and nurtured particularly by the Summer Institutes on Integration originated by the Canadian Association for Community Living (CACL) and McGill University. These institutes now take place across the country because of partnerships between universities and CACL. The newly formed Centre for Integrated Education and Community is active in the education of professionals and consultation with local school boards.

Changes in provincial legislation, local initiatives, the experience and expertise of professionals, and the authority of the Canadian Charter of Rights and Freedoms provide an increasingly effective and diverse set of tools to be used in promoting full integration and inclusion. Thus, in contrast to the traditional pattern of segregated services, intervention, early childhood, and public education programs in a growing number of communities across Canada are enabling a generation of children with and without specified special needs to grow up together as friends and learners.

ISRAEL

In Israel compulsory free education is provided for all children from age 5 to 18. In addition, over 80% of children ages 3 and 4 attend public or private nursery school programs. Education is the responsibility of local government agencies, with the Ministry of Education providing funding, a standard curriculum, teacher training, and matriculation examinations. In addition, the kibbutz movement and various religious groups operate publicly funded separate school systems.

The Ministry's Unit for Special Education has the responsibility for education of children with disabilities, except children with severe mental disabilities, whose education is the responsibility of the Ministry of Labor and Social Welfare. The

Unit also provides vocational training for adolescents with disabilities until the age of 18.

In 1976, the Ministry of Education and Culture issued a special bylaw providing a new definition of the special child. This bylaw provided that any assessment of the child must be functional and not categorical, and must be based upon a detailed analysis of the cognitive, physical, and emotional functioning of the child along with recommendations for a rehabilitation plan. A new special education law, passed in 1988, extended educational services for children with disabilities through age 21. This law also introduced a provision that allows parents the right to appeal the educational placement offered to their child. Parents can also play a role in enhancing and expanding the activities of the special education system through a nationwide parent committee for special education.

The majority of the child developmental clinics, described in Chapter 5, conduct programs for preschool age children with disabilities. While there is considerable attention to the importance of parental involvement in the development and education of their children, no national policy mandates their involvement. There are, however, efforts by various parent organizations to develop parent involvement programs on the local level.

Parent training is well established in the areas of visual and auditory impairments. Home teachers are an important government service for children with visual impairments. These teachers, in addition to direct instruction of the child, work with the family in the home. Parents are provided instruction in how to meet the special developmental needs of their child. For children with hearing impairments, regional centers established by MICHA, a parent-organized voluntary group, provide services for children from birth through 6 years of age. Services are provided both at the MICHA centers and in the family's home.

Voluntary groups also provide similar services. For example, AKIM (mentioned in Chapter 5) has trained community rehabilitation teachers to work in the homes of children with physical disabilities and to provide training and support for families. The Rehabilitation Center and Nursery School at Cholim Hospital in Jerusalem provides a similar program. At Bar-Ilan University, there is a systematic program for training parents of children with developmental disabilities, conducted in cooperation with various parent organizations. An innovative project in the School of Education at Tel Aviv University trains parents to support their children in their home.

JAPAN

In Japan all children ages 6–15 are entitled to a free school education, regardless of the nature and severity of any disability. Prefectural governments are required to provide special schools for children with mental disabilities, emotional disturbances, and for those with physical disabilities; the schools are organized by category of disability, for example, blindness, deafness, loss of limbs, and so forth. While some children with disabilities are integrated into regular school classes, the great majority of children with disabilities attend either special schools or special classes in regular schools. Children with speech impairments are taught in regular classes, attending special speech sessions; there are visiting teachers for children who remain at home or in residential facilities. And there are schools attached to residential facilities and hospitals. A limited amount of vocational education is provided to students with disabilities by the special schools at the junior and senior high school levels.

Day-care centers for children with different impairments are authorized by the Child Welfare Law, and the national government provides some subsidies. In small communities where size precludes the operation of separate programs for children with different handicapping conditions, combined services are offered to children regardless of the type of impairment. The centers provide weekday services for children 3 years of age and older who are able to attend for the full week. Generally, children with more severe impairments and those under age 3 are kept at home, although some programs have begun to serve these children. Many of the day-care programs require maternal participation. The expectation is that the mothers will learn how to care for and provide appropriate stimulation to their children. Despite the legal requirement for such programs, many communities do not provide services. In Yokohama, for example, in the absence of public services, more than 25 parent groups conduct such programs.

Habilitation and rehabilitation services in Japan are provided on both residential and nonresidential bases for children with disabilities, and the facilities are categorically organized.

KENYA

In Kenya national legislation provides for universal education. It is not yet, however, available throughout the country, especially in the rural areas in which the majority of the population lives. This is particularly true for students with disabilities.

The Ministry of Health and the Ministry of Education operate assessment centres in each province and provide parent education. In many areas of the country, however, the absence of publicly provided education leaves children with disabilities on their own, without needed services or assistance. The Civitan Foundation, a private organization, provides parent workshops in cooperation with the Ministry of Health and Education. The network of district hospitals is also an important resource in developing parent education programs.

SWEDEN

In Sweden 9 years of schooling are compulsory for all children starting at age 7. Over 90% of youth go on to at least 2 years of upper secondary schooling, choosing from among a variety of vocational or academic tracks. Schools are run by municipalities and provide free instruction, books, and lunches. The special school is part of the local community school, but offered through special classes. Every child from a non-Swedish speaking home over the age of 5 has the right to four lessons a week in her or his native language.

Parent involvement is considered essential. For children with disabilities under age seven, a special teacher either visits the child's home or provides services at the local community preschool. All children with disabilities between the ages of 2 and 7 are integrated in the local preschool. Therapy services, as necessary, are provided on a similar basis, with assistance as well to the parents to encourage their involvement.

THE UNITED KINGDOM

In the United Kingdom, each of the 120 Local Authorities includes a Local Education Authority (LEA) that is responsible for all education services (except universities) for both children and adults. The 1944 Educational Act was the first to require LEAs to meet the needs of students with disabilities within their general duties to provide primary and secondary education. During the 1950s and 1960s, the issue of education for children with disabilities became one of a number of concerns within a broad commitment to equal opportunities; the Warnock Report in 1978 recommended a new and much broader definition of special education needs and a much closer partnership with parents.

The 1981 Education Act is perhaps the most significant piece of legislation in the UK specifically targeted at children and youth with special needs. In large part, it was based upon the recommendations of the Warnock Committee on the Education of Handicapped Children and Young People. The Committee adopted an expansive definition of special education needs, noting that at any given time one child in six was likely to have such needs. The Committee used the term "learning difficulties" to describe a child who has a "significantly greater difficulty in learning than the majority of children of his [sic] age or has a disability which either prevents or hinders . . . him from making use of educational facilities of a kind generally provided in schools . . . for children of his age." Thus, the 1981 legislation at a stroke expanded the number of children to be served from the previous 2% in special schools to a much larger number—as much as 20%, in ordinary schools. The legislation places a statutory duty on the governors of all schools to identify and meet the special education needs of each of their pupils. Furthermore, the legislation requires educational authorities to work with: 1) local health and social services to identify a child's needs and 2) parents to provide information, participate in assessment, and develop a program to meet the child's special education needs. While the language of the act concerning parental involvement is broadly framed, in practice it is concerned with that group of parents whose children are having a formal "statement" of need developed, that is, all children in special schools and those children in ordinary schools for whom additional services are needed. For this group, the act lays down a number of important parental rights and safeguards: 1) to participate in discussions and decision-making, 2) to prepare written documents and other evidence, 3) to have access to an officer of the LEA and to see certain documents, and 4) to appeal to the LEA and as a last resort to the Secretary of State.

The 1978 Warnock Report, noted above, which was the first UK government report to address seriously the possibility of partnership with parents in the education of their children, stated that the relationship between parents and professionals

> should be a partnership and ideally an equal one . . . for although we tend to dwell upon the dependence of many parents on professional support, we are well aware that professional help cannot be wholly effective, if at all so, unless it builds upon the parents' capacity to be involved. . . . [P]arents can be effective partners only if professionals take notice of what they say and of how they express their needs and treat their contribution as intrinsically important. (*Special education needs,* 1978, p. 83)

The principles of partnership with parents were built into the assessment procedures of the 1981 Education Act, with parents given new rights and duties with regard to contributing to decision-making about their children. A 1987 House of Commons Select Committee Report indicates that the rhetoric remains stronger than the reality, however.

Despite the anxieties raised by the Select Committee, among school personnel there is growing awareness of the need to involve parents and the need for greater sensitivity concerning how such participation may be organized. From the 1960s onward, there has been increasing involvement of parents in early education, with the recognition that the family is the most effective and economical system for fostering and sustaining the development of a young child. Studies among families with children with Down syndrome and other studies looking more broadly at early educational experiences report that good early education including support for families makes families as well as children more confident and competent and more adaptable to subsequent opportunities and services.

A number of early years home visiting programs have been developed in the UK, ranging from Homestart, which provides primarily parent support, with developmental activities for the child, through trained, usually volunteer home visitors, to Portage. Portage, which originated in the United States, has had a powerful impact on professional thinking in the UK about the potential of parents as educators of young children with special needs. (For more information on the Portage Model for Home Teaching see Paine, Bellamy, & Wilcox, 1984.)

The central feature of the Portage home teaching process is that the home teachers and parents together identify and agree upon new skills that they would like to see the child with special needs acquire. Working together, they develop appropriate methods of teaching these skills. The parents receive assistance in understanding their child's existing skills, selecting objectives that build upon the child's current skills, and participating in a program individualized for their child that enables the parents to be successful with her or him. A growing number of schools are developing programs based upon the Portage model and are developing parent support groups to provide extended opportunities for parents not only to understand their own child, but also to understand the complex network of health, education, and social services that may be necessary to achieve desired goals.

A number of Local Authorities have begun a process of parental involvement by conducting surveys on what parents actually want. The parents' responses were remarkably similar in all Local Authorities. Priorities included: clearer information, with an acknowledgment that the process of assessment may be painful; a desire to be referred to relevant voluntary organizations that could give support, advice, and companionship; clearer policies; fewer delays in assessments; and a desire for assistance in the assessment process. The Warnock Commission's recommendations that all parents whose children are going through the assessment process have a "named person" or advocate to guide and assist them was given high priority. The Department of Education and Science has given a 3-year grant to the Voluntary Council for Handicapped Children to identify, develop, and disseminate information on a range of initiatives to help parents in becoming partners and to take account of families who have other special needs, such as families from minority ethnic groups.

Many parent groups are directly involved with Local Educational Authorities in producing "user friendly" information and in developing a range of forums and other opportunities for parents to meet, befriend, and join in advocacy with other parents. One major scheme is SNAP (Special Needs Advisory Project) in South Wales, where three national voluntary organizations have joined with three education departments to recruit, train, and support a number of volunteer parent "befrienders" who would help other parents during assessment. The KIDS Centre, in Camden, London has developed a similar scheme for younger children, drawing its befrienders from the local community and providing training and support. Several voluntary organizations have provided professional befrienders.

The 1981 Education Act stipulates that the child with special education needs should be educated in ordinary schools, provided that: the child receives the special education services she or he needs, "efficient education" can be provided for other pupils, there is "efficient" use of resources, "functional integration" is "reasonably practical," and account has been taken of the parents' wishes. While progress in integration has been mixed, the concept of integration as a process is reflected in an increasing trend toward part-time integration; that is, students who attend special schools attend local regular schools part time, with the special school staff supporting the activities at the regular school. Although there is a general move toward integration, significant numbers of children continue to attend special schools or units that have greater resources than do mainstream schools. (For further treatment of these issues, see Barton, 1988.)

Young people have the right to further education up to the age of 19. The special needs of special education students continue at a secondary school. Some colleges provide special programs and access to integrated courses for students with special needs.

The 1988 Education Reform Act offers further opportunities for—and poses potential threats to—children with special education needs in the United Kingdom. The act aims to "promote the spiritual, moral, cultural, mental, and physical development of pupils" through the introduction of a national curriculum. Guidelines for the act indicate that the "Curriculum is expected to be balanced and broadly based and relevant to the full range of pupils' needs." Further, it is noted that "The Secretary of State believes that all pupils, including those with special education needs, should have the opportunity to obtain the maximum benefit possible from it." Section 2 of the act sets out the arrangements for the national curriculum, including attainment targets, programs of study, and assessment arrangements. Each of the core subjects are to be taught according to the specified attainment targets, programs of study, and assessment arrangements during the four stages of compulsory education, from ages 5 through 16 years. Variations are permitted for individual students who may progress at different rates through the programs of study. Exemptions to the national curriculum are to be made on a temporary basis by the Head Teacher, subject to certain conditions and open to appeal, or through modification to the statement developed for each child with special educational needs.

In principle, children with special education needs may have greater access to a wider curriculum. However, there is a growing concern among some in the UK that schools, which now are acquiring new responsibilities for managing their finances, may be reluctant to give priority to special needs students. Furthermore, the requirement to publish data as to student achievement may lead some schools to feel that these students will spoil their records. On the positive side, parents will have available to them information on how their child is progressing, and Statements of Special Educational Needs should become more explicit about the sort of curriculum that is needed to help a particular child. The 1988 Act complements the 1981 Act. Given the growing pressure for formal assessment and statements that provide for rights to services and commitments of resources, local authorities may be loath to make commitments until a formal and complex assessment procedure is completed, thus delaying the provision of special education.

No single authority has overall responsibility for services for children under 5 years of age. Thus, services vary widely from jurisdiction to jurisdiction. Among the services offered are home-based programs, home liaison or advisory teachers, organized play or opportunity groups often run by voluntary organizations, day nurseries frequently operated by local social services agencies, and nursery schools or classes with special arrangements for children with disabilities operated by education authorities.

THE UNITED STATES OF AMERICA

In the United States of America providing children with an education is the responsibility of each state. Beginning in the nineteenth century, some school systems and states provided services for some children with handicapping conditions. By the middle of the twentieth century, most states offered programs for some children with handicaps. Sparked by the school desegregation cases of the 1950s, parents of children with disabilities brought a series of court suits challenging the exclusion of children with disabilities from educational services or the provision of less than equal services to them. At the same time, the federal government began to provide limited funding for certain education programs, including education for students with handicapping conditions. With the passage of PL 94-142, The Education for All Handicapped Children Act of 1975, each state that sought federal support was required: 1) to provide a free and appropriate education for all children, regardless of the nature and severity of their impairments; 2) to identify and certify as handicapped and in need of special education services only those children who were evaluated through a multidisciplinary and nondiscriminatory assessment procedure; 3) to provide individually appropriate services in the least restrictive environment; and 4) to ensure parental due process rights in the assessment of, planning for, and delivery of services to the child. Initially, the law covered children from age 5 through age 21. In 1986, amendments to the law (PL 99-457, the Education of the Handicapped Act Amendments) extended its coverage to include children from birth to 5 years of age, the infants and toddlers. In these programs, the Individualized Education Program (IEP) of PL 94-142 is replaced by an Individualized Family Service Plan (IFSP) for each child and family served. As with PL 94-142, each of the 50 states has opted to participate in this program. Funding is provided predominantly by state and local governments, with the federal contribution below 10%.

In many ways, the implementation of PL 94-142 has been a major achievement, particularly in terms of providing access to needed services. Less successful have been efforts to ensure positive outcomes, that is, student benefit as reflected in subsequent employment, education, or community living (Gartner & Lipsky, 1989). Currently, there is a growing debate about the direction of special education in the United States. Key in this debate has been consideration of the integration of students with handicapping conditions into regular classrooms. A number of states and school districts are pursuing full integration for students, which has been the topic of considerable attention. (For further information on integration see Lipsky & Gartner, 1989; Sailor et al., 1989; and Stainback, Stainback, & Forest, 1989.)

In the United States, there is great reliance upon professionals to provide systematic instruction and specialized interventions to persons with disabilities. During the 1970s and 1980s, great effort has been exerted to study the utility of particular training and habilitation techniques to promote efficient skill acquisition and parental education. As a result, many instructional materials are available tailored to the needs of the parents and individual child; taking into account the child's age and nature and severity of impairment; and often focusing on particular instructional needs (e.g., community living skills, self-help skills, early development stages). Another area where considerable work has been done is the development of instructional strategies that serve to promote integration (e.g., cooperative learning, peer tutoring, special friends).

Additionally, there is increasing attention being paid to studies of family life, both in terms of involvement in instructional activities and in understanding the consequences and effects of having a child with a disability. Strategies to facilitate skill acquisition at home continue to evolve, with three issues receiving great attention: what to teach, how to teach, and the family's role in shaping the service delivery process.

URUGUAY

In Uruguay services for students with disabilities have followed a pattern of first struggle for inclusion and later efforts to achieve integration. Beginning in the middle of the twentieth century, first private and then public programs were established for students with disabilities. In 1961 the Department of Special Education was established at the national level. In the following two decades, increasing numbers of students with disabilities were served, largely in separate settings. Since the mid-1980s, there has been a shift from segregation to integration and a more participatory approach. A Restructuring Plan adopted in 1986 provides for pilot plans to: 1) integrate students with disabilities into the regular curriculum at the elementary and vocational school level, 2) create support teachers at regular schools, 3) develop a center for attention to student psychiatric problems, 4) organize work centers for students with severe and profound handicaps, 5) integrate the education of students with hearing impairments, and 6) establish a postgraduate teacher education center.

CONCLUSION

For the family of a child with disabilities, education is many things. First, of course, it provides the child with the means to live a productive life. Also education is an aspect of participating in society. In terms of the effect of the child's education on the family, when the child attends school— especially with her or his age peers—the family is seen less as "special," more as "normal." And, as with all families, the child's time in school frees family members from care responsibilities, providing them general relief and the opportunity to pursue their own activities.

REFERENCES

Barton, L. (Ed.). (1988). *The politics of special education needs.* London: The Falmer Press.

Gartner, A., & Lipsky, D.K. (1989, June). *Equity and excellence.* Presentation before the National Council of Disability, National Study of the Education of Students with Disabilities, Washington, D.C.

Lipsky, D.K., & Gartner, A. (Eds.). (1989). *Beyond separate education: Quality education for all.* Baltimore: Paul H. Brookes Publishing Co.

Paine, S.C., Bellamy, G. T., & Wilcox, B. (Eds.). (1984). *Human services that work: From innovation to standard practice.* Baltimore: Paul H. Brookes Publishing Co.

Sailor, W.A., Anderson, J.L., Halvorsen, A.T., Doering, K., Filler, J., & Goetz, L. (Eds.). (1989). *The comprehensive local school: Regular education for all students with disabilities.* Baltimore: Paul H. Brookes Publishing Co.

Special education needs. (1978). London: Her Majesty's Stationery Office.

Stainback, S., Stainback, W., & Forest, M. (Eds.). (1989). *Educating all students in the mainstream of regular education.* Baltimore: Paul H. Brookes Publishing Co.

7

Taking a Break from Responsibility for Meeting the Child's Needs

The framing or formulation of the issue of taking a break from responsibility for meeting the needs of a child with a disability, which in a number of countries is called "respite," is of major consequence. One aspect of this issue was noted in Chapter 2 where the basic understanding of disability, the distinction between impairment and handicap, as well as the cultural meanings of disability were discussed. The question here is whether what is commonly called "respite" is seen as an opportunity for the nondisabled family members to take a break from responsibility for the needs of the child with a disability or an opportunity for the child with a disability to be in and gain from a different setting and/or to be with other people. The first need can be met by various alternative arrangements in the child's home or elsewhere. To the extent that the second need is valued, a different set of circumstances must be addressed. As this chapter indicates, it is possible to incorporate both of these goals into the family's situation, or at least to seek a balance between them.[1]

---

[1]The balance (or tension) between these formulations of the issue is also seen in services for adults with disabilities. Several recent publications of the World Institute on Disability have addressed this topic. (See especially Litvak, Zukas, & Heumann, 1987.)

Current formulations of the issue, as reflected in the language used, however, do not reflect this balance. Rather, "respite" generally is seen from the perspective of the needs of nondisabled family members for a break from caring for the child with a disability. Such relief may better enable the nondisabled family members to meet the needs of the child.

Respite services provided for this purpose are viewed as an adjunct to the basic services that the child may receive. Indeed, basic service provision to the child with a disability is itself a form of respite. That is, for example, while the child attends school the family is relieved of direct care responsibilities and at the same time the child receives direct benefits.

As is true in the services described in the previous chapters, there is considerable variety among the nine countries in respite care. This is the case, however, within the context of a common framing of the issue from the perspective of the nondisabled family members. That is, respite is provided to aid the nondisabled family members.

There is variety not only in the ways in which respite is provided but also in the extent to which the need for respite services is seen as something unique only to families with a child with a disability. Furthermore, there is variety in the extent to which this need is to be met as a social service system function or as a part of natural kin and friendship networks.

For the purposes of the discussion here, respite is understood as an occasional short-term activity that takes place when in its absence the child would be cared for by a family member. A different set of issues, beyond the scope of our analysis here, concerns the arrangements necessary to enable adult family members to obtain employment or to obtain an education.[2]

GENERAL ARRANGEMENTS

In six of the nine countries (Australia, Canada, Japan, Sweden, the United Kingdom, and the United States of America), there

---

[2]For a study of such arrangements in the United States, see Krauskopf and Akabas (1988). The most interesting datum, in an admittedly preliminary survey, is "there was . . . no significant difference in . . . work pattern for families with a disabled child as compared with families in which the newborn had no identified disability" (p. 31).

are government provided (or supported) respite activities. In Australia and Japan some of the respite programs are provided by the national government. In Israel, a few private organizations provide respite services. There are not formal respite services in Kenya or Uruguay, although some residential service agencies on occasion make "beds" available.

AUSTRALIA

In Australia the focus of respite arrangements is on short-term relief for people whose long-term support arrangements, in its absence, would be at risk. Priority, under the Disability Services Act of 1986, is given to children with intensive care needs. While this act provides for out-of-home respite, under the Home and Community Care Act of 1985 in-home respite may be provided, either as a primary service or as an outcome of the provision of home help or personal care.

Out-of-home services are provided through use of beds in existing institutional settings, a decreasing alternative, and increasingly through specific respite houses, as well as through host families who are recruited, trained, and paid to provide short periods of respite.

CANADA

In Canada too, there is a shift from the use of beds in institutional settings to greater use of community-based arrangements. These include: 1) respite families, who serve the same function as beds in residences except in a family setting (in some instances, this has become a form of specialized foster care); 2) respite workers, hired by a local government or private agency, to come into the child's home; and 3) extend-a-family arrangements. In one variant of extend-a-family programs families are recruited and paid by the government to have the child with a disability for a day or overnight or to visit longer. Another variant of respite encourages friendships between families, facilitated by a paid coordinator who recruits, matches, and supports pairings of families. Other community arrangements include: 1) associate family arrangements, which involve more intensive relationships that range from short-term visits to having the child with a disability living for protracted periods with the associate family and visiting his or her own family on a regular basis; and 2) government supported programs that hire individuals to provide direct services to the child with a disability, with one of the benefits being that the family has a break.

ISRAEL

In Israel only a few parent or community organizations provide respite services. Indeed, their absence, it is reported, leads many parents to institutionalize their children with severe mental handicaps. AKIM, an organization developed by parents to serve children with multihandicaps, established the first respite care services at several of its branches. In the Arab community, the extended family is seen as the natural supplier of respite services.

JAPAN

In Japan since 1970 national legislation has provided home help services to persons with physical disabilities, both children and adults. A secondary benefit of these services, which are also provided by some local authorities, is respite.

In Yokohama, the Society for Disabled Persons' Community Living subsidizes the transportation costs of respite volunteers, who are usually recruited by the families who have a child with a disability. The volunteers do such things as take the children to and from needed services when the parents are unavailable, help the children with their homework, or spend an afternoon with the child.

KENYA

In Kenya there are no organized respite services for the family. In the rural areas—that is 80% of the country, where tribal bonds remain strong—members of the extended family or clan may offer assistance. In the growing urban area, where families are more isolated, such supports are less available and families either leave a child unattended or a family member must always be available.

SWEDEN

In Sweden the county councils provide respite services through short-term homes or relief families. After families are matched, if they find confidence in and compatibility with each other, a formal program is established. At that time, relief families receive supervision and training through the local government. Non-Swedish families are less likely to use such formal respite services, preferring a relative who speaks the language and knows the customs.

THE UNITED KINGDOM

In the United Kingdom respite or short-term care services for families with a disabled child have developed historically as emergency services. Frequently such services were provided through a hospital or other institutional setting, often at a considerable distance from the family's home. Although the early forms of respite were often offered in "block" bookings for summer holidays or similar periods, services have now become much more flexible and many families can have respite care provision on demand. The objectives of respite care are now seen as providing a local service, whereby the child can continue to attend school as if he or she were living at home, and where good quality child care is the primary concern. Although some children still receive respite care in a hospital or in a Local Authority or voluntary children's home, the majority receive such services through substitutive family care. There are now over 50 family-based respite care programs in the United Kingdom and a national organization of such programs was launched in 1989. Substitute families are recruited locally and receive training, support, and payment through the Local Authority or voluntary organization running the program. Parents with children with disabilities usually can use the service on demand, and close friendships are often formed.

Despite these gains, however, there is general recognition of the need to continue the development of respite care services. Many families with children with multiple disabilities or major behavior disorders have difficulty finding help. And one study (Robinson, 1988) points out that respite should not be seen as a total solution but as an integral part of an overall family plan for support services.

Other studies have highlighted particular concerns; for example, the fact that many families have no knowledge of respite services, the anxiety for some families of leaving their child overnight, the need for more flexible and short-term (several hours) respite. But despite problems, the availability of respite care is growing; this increasing availability has been associated with parental willingness to continue to care for children with severe disabilities in the community. Many of the new generation of successful adoptive and long-term foster parents of children with a range of disabilities have also emphasized the importance of respite care in enabling them to continue to cope. There has been no comparative research on parental satisfaction with different models of respite care, but it seems that parents are likely to use services and be more satisfied if they feel the service is good for the child and if the service offered is local, accessible, and linked to other service outlets, such as school, a child development center, or a voluntary organization.

THE UNITED STATES OF AMERICA

In the United States of America beginning in the early 1970s, the growing commitment to a community-centered response to the needs of persons with disabilities has prompted increased demand from parents for respite services. While originally conceived of as a way of preventing long-term, out-of-home placement of children, it has become clear that respite could lead to improvement of family functioning by giving parents an opportunity to rest, to spend time with each other, to attend to the needs of their other children, to visit with friends, or to be alone. Despite the recognized benefits of these functions, most publicly supported respite care arrangements continue to have a narrow focus.

Respite care services in the United States take many forms. They may be provided in the family home, in the home of the provider, or at a service center. They may be provided for a few hours, several days, or even for a couple of weeks. They may be provided by a teenager with a brief training course, by a volunteer family that receives orientation from the parents, by another family with a child with a disability in an exchange relationship or cooperative, by a respite care worker trained and employed by a public or private agency, or by a health care professional. While the variety of arrangements is considerable, the actual availability of services is far more limited. And in any given location the particular type of service a family may need— in-home versus out-of-home, for example—may not be available.

A survey sent to readers of *Exceptional Parent* reinforces these points and adds others (Knoll & Bedford, 1989a, 1989b). While those who utilize respite services find them valuable, there are problems in terms of "lack of flexibility, arbitrary limits on the use of the service, the inability of the service system to respond to crises. . ." (Knoll & Bedford, 1989b, p. 34). Parents want to be in control of the service, and have the provider of the service responsible to them. They prefer someone they know, or failing that, someone who is understood to be their employee. Despite the understanding of respite services as community-based and family-centered, Knoll and Bedford conclude:

> We found little evidence that the respite system has truly left behind the traditional professional-client relationship. There is no clear evidence that the majority of respite programs are consistent with the values of consumer empowerment and control. If there were consistency, we would expect to find substantive consumer involvement in the design, management, and evaluation of support services. We did not. (p. 37)

A growing development, similar to that in Canada, is the rediscovery of the informal human resources that surround families. An as yet small but increasing number of programs are learning to use public funds to strengthen informal support networks, with families being asked to identify individuals among their relatives and friends to be trained to provide respite care.

URUGUAY

In Uruguay several of the large residential facilities provide respite as an ancillary activity. These include a home for persons with mental retardation and a school for persons with visual impairments. Also, the national school for the deaf has established a network of foster homes that occasionally provide respite services.

ISSUES AND PROBLEMS

In each of the countries, regardless of the nature or extent of the program, there is the belief that what is available both falls far short of general need and often does not respond to the individual circumstances and needs of families or children. This applies to issues such as the type of arrangements, that is, in-home versus out-of-home; their appropriateness for the child in terms of age, impairment, and level of development; the times when services are available, with particular gaps during evenings, weekends, and holidays; the frequency with which services may be used; and the need for advanced planning versus on demand arrangements. Added to these issues is the question of the quality of the services provided.

The availability of institutional settings, many of which are less utilized as more community-based living arrangements are developed, makes them an apparently attractive option for respite. Issues to be addressed here, however, include the extent to which this disrupts the lives of the facility's residents, the potential for the child to learn inappropriate behaviors from others in such settings (although this could occur either way), the child being with strangers, the often restrictive regulations in such facilities, and the possibility (and fear) that an arrangement for short-term relief might become one of long-term care.

The major current developments for respite involve government provided (or supported) respite services, with given jurisdictions offering a particular type (or occasionally types) of services. Given the range of family circumstances and needs, a more appropriate design would involve a cafeteria of services from which a family could choose the appropriate arrangement at a given time. A further extension of this would give the family the power and resources to choose (or establish) the arrangements best suited to it, either through a cash allowance or voucher scheme. Even within a pre-existing arrangement, giving the family the authority to hire, supervise, and pay the respite care worker would increase the family's autonomy and strengthen its coping capacity.

Regardless of the organizational issues, there is the matter of the cultural appropriateness of such services. Clearly, persons who speak the family's language and know its rules and customs are more likely to be used and provide better services.

CONCLUSION

Successful respite services are offered in diverse ways. In all of the countries studied there appears to be agreement that respite services, formal or informal, are essential for families. The broad issues are the ones with which we began this chapter: the purposes for which respite is to be provided; the perspective from which respite is to be provided, that is, the family's or the child's; the relationship of respite to other services the family may require; and the integration of respite into the larger sphere of the family's life. The needs of the child with a disability and those of other family members, while they may overlap, are not identical. Thus, if we are to talk about a system of respite, it must offer the potential to meet the different, as well as common needs of each of the parties. Some arrangements can do both, while others, appropriately, meet the needs of one or the other.

The growing attention to connecting respite services to so-called informal support services—for example, allowing families to identify friends and relatives to be engaged as respite providers—is a welcome development. However, there is the danger that what in other circumstances would be a normal development—for example, taking a friend's child (who happens to have a disability) to a ball game—could become a social service and, in effect, turn friendship into a commodity.

REFERENCES

Knoll, J.A., & Bedford, S. (1989a). *Becoming informed consumers: A national survey of parents' experience with respite services.* Cambridge, MA: Human Services Research Institute.

Knoll, J., & Bedford, S. (1989b). Respite services: A national survey of parents' experience. *Exceptional Parent, 19*(4), 34–37.

Krauskopf, M.S., & Akabas, S.H. (1988). Children with disabilities: A family/workplace partnership in problem resolution. *Social Work Papers, XXI,* 28–35.

Litvak, S.L., Zukas, H., & Heumann, J.E. (1987). *Attending to America. Personal assistance for independent living.* Berkeley: World Institute on Disability.

Robinson, C. (1988). *Avon short-term respite care scheme: An evaluation study.* Bristol, U.K.: University of Bristol.

8

Emotional Support

Emotional support, of course, is something that all people need to help make sense of their circumstances and keep themselves going. In principle, this is no more—and no less—the case for families with a child with a disability than it is for any other family. It becomes a matter of special concern in the context of what the society does. This is so both in terms of how it teaches the parents (both explicitly and, more consequentially, implicitly through the broader message concerning the view of disability, as discussed in Chapter 2) to understand, interpret, and respond to the child and her or his impairment and in the nature of the supports it provides. The presence of a child with a disability can be a blessing, a burden, both, or neither of these, some or all of the time. The same is true of the presence of a child without a disability. Which of these situations is the case and how they are responded to is not always given. It is an individual matter set in the context of societal framing. Too often, just as the child with an impairment becomes the impairment (e.g., a boy with spina bifida is referred to as the spina bifida boy), so too, the family is labeled. And with this label comes a set of assumptions about capacity, or more usually incapacity. In turn, these assumptions affect the nature of the response to the family's situation. For example, if the family of a child with disabilities is seen as inevitably overcome by emotional problems and trauma unique to the situation of having the child, then the response identified as appropriate is a set of psychological services geared to this unique situation. If, however, it is understood that families—those with and those without a child with a disability—are more alike than different and all families have the need for emotional support, then the supports identified for them are both general and specific but not pathology oriented. Thus, emotional support becomes something that is not uniquely a need of families with a child with a disability; rather, it is something that all families need. How that need manifests itself and the ways to respond to it will vary family by family along a wide range of factors, only one of which is whether there is a child with a disability in the family. We use this framework to examine the ways in which the nine countries provide emotional support to meet the needs of families with a child with a disability.

Furthermore, the framework relates to understanding the need for emotional support within the context of meeting the full range of the family's needs. The extent to which there is stress and consequentially a need for a particular type of emotional support is a function of the interaction between the burdens placed upon the family system and the resources provided both to address the burdens and to support the family. Thus, for example, the consequence for the family of a child who is chronically incontinent is different in the presence or absence of a washing machine. And the availability of a circle of friends, while it does not change the child's impairment, does have consequence for the impact upon the family, both the stress it bears and the resources it brings to that circumstance. The very concept that it is friends who are needed or, indeed, who are appropriate, in contrast to the traditional call for service providers, is in itself a factor in assessing a family's needs for emotional support and the ways to provide it.

AUSTRALIA

In Australia there is no formal system whereby families can gain emotional support either in dealing with the meaning of giving birth to a child with a disability or in meeting the ongoing emotional needs of the family. Emotional support is provided either by peer support through parent groups or by professionals to whom parents and other family members may be referred.

Australia's history of high dependence on service-providing voluntary agencies had led to a greater involvement of parents in service provision as opposed to advocacy or parent support. Parent support is usually voluntary and consists of parents of children with specific disabilities coming together and being available to other parents. Typically, these groups will produce leaflets or newsletters and advertise themselves in hospitals, doctors' offices, and baby health centers. Some parent groups have become more formally organized and may receive limited support from local governments.

There are few funded parent support groups at the state or regional levels. Some parent-to-parent programs have been established at these levels whereby individual parents are recruited and trained to offer emotional support to other parents. When children with disabilities reach school age, emotional support is often an offshoot of meeting other parents at school associations. Professional emotional support is most often gained through the social workers at hospitals or through regional developmental disability teams.

CANADA

In Canada there is an array of traditional and formal sources and types of emotional support. Increasingly, however, the need for emotional support is coming to be viewed in the context of challenging the view that families with a child with a disability have the experience of a dream denied because a less-than-perfect child has entered their family. There is a focus upon enabling the family to regain the ability to dream, to create a vision of the present and future that is fundamentally similar to their dreams for other members of the family.

Thus, in Canada a growing body of information and activity reinterprets the meaning of disability and tells positive stories about people with disabilities bringing their talents to bear on the lives of other individuals and the community, and about communities welcoming these talents. So too, there is a growing corps of professionals whose job it is to assist families in thinking about what they need. These supports are most evident in situations of family crisis or changes in public policy such as deinstitutionalization efforts, when immediate and systematic action is required. To a lesser extent, these supports are beginning to be offered in planning services for young people leaving school.

There is increasing availability of funding for families to fulfill their own dreams by purchasing services from or through agencies responsive to their individual situations. Additionally, in some places and in some circumstances families are gaining increasing control over plans and actions, which are developed for them, occasionally with them, and sometimes by them. Service experience is expanding with the development of individual service planning, program planning, individual education plans, and the like for the purpose of responding to individual desires as opposed to agency determinations. And there are a growing number of groups and networks forming to support individuals, mostly adults but sometimes school age children, and free them to dream and to focus on the question of what they really want for their lives.

ISRAEL

In Israel there are two main sources of emotional support for parents of a child with a disability. First is the formal support provided by a number of government and parent organizations. However, these have no defined policy concerning how, when, and by whom emotional support is provided.

Second, there are the services provided to the parents of a child with a disability by various community resources: social workers in maternity and neonatal departments, public health nurses in the mother and child clinics, and staff members in the centers for child development. For children with specific impairments, there are individually organized parent support groups. A joint project of the Tel-Aviv district health office and the Department of Nursing of Tel-Aviv University trains public health nurses in meeting the needs of children with a chronic illness and how to work with their families. Beit Izzie Shapiro has a special unit where parents of children with a mental disability can receive counseling and emotional support. And the School for Parents of Children with a Developmental Disability was set up to offer the parents an opportunity to learn skills and obtain emotional support. As children grow up and participate in a preschool program, the parents may be able to receive counseling and support from the professionals in that setting. There are also self-help groups available that have been established by voluntary parent organizations, such as AKIM, NITZAN, MICHA, and SHEMA (which were mentioned in Chapter 5). The number of these groups has increased in the 1980s, and there are now over 20 such groups in Israel. Among the kibbutz movement, self-help groups have been formed among parents of children with a disability to increase emotional support. Among the Arab population, emotional support is generally informal and provided mostly by members of the extended family. In the 1980s an attempt was begun to coordinate such efforts for families in general and particularly for Arab children with disabilities and their families in the Nazareth area.

JAPAN

In Japan the Welfare Laws for the Physically Disabled and for the Mentally Disabled stipulate that public health centers, child guidance centers, and welfare offices are to be the focal points of information and services in the community for children with disabilities and their families. During the early years of the child's life, public health nurses at the public health centers and at the local authorities' maternal and child health centers are key resources. New parents of children with disabilities are encouraged to participate as observers in small play groups organized by these nurses as a way to learn about the conditions of children with disabilities, to ask questions, and to provide a basis for coming to terms with their children's conditions.

Parents' groups are seen as important sources of information and emotional support. Associations of parents of children with mental retardation and children with physical disabilities were formed in the early 1950s. Additional groups among parents with children with other disabilities were organized in subsequent decades. These groups provide both emotional support for their members and act as a pressure group to improve the services available to their children. In addition to the mutual support activities among the members of these groups, some local welfare offices have recruited experienced parents of children with disabilities to work with and provide emotional support to new parents.

KENYA

In Kenya tribal and kinship networks are both elaborate and extensive and form a basis for the provision of services that otherwise (and elsewhere) might be offered by governments. The birth of a child is something that affects not only the parents and immediate family but the entire clan. Thus, the joy, or sadness, that this evokes is widespread. Whatever the response—while it varies both between tribes and among individuals—the family and the clan are the sources of support, both physical and emotional. These efforts serve to knit more closely an already intimate system of reciprocal support.

Having a child with a disability is most often viewed as a tragedy. In some circumstances, the negative response is such that the family not only denies the existence of the child, they seek to hide the child. In such circumstances the support of family or clan is precluded, and the parents become even further isolated; this is particularly the case when families have moved into urban areas where traditional forms of support are limited.

SWEDEN

In Sweden the major service-provision activities are available through the county councils. For example, the County Council of Stockholm, the nation's largest unit, has a special team of psychologists and social workers who provide psychotherapy to parents of children with disabilities. They provide individual therapy, or work with couples, or in small groups. This support is available free. However, the absence of therapists who speak languages other than Swedish in the employ of the county councils precludes such services to non–Swedish speaking families other than through an interpreter, since the government insurance programs do not reimburse families when they must find a psychologist not employed by a county council.

THE UNITED KINGDOM

In the United Kingdom the majority of service providers for families with a young child with a disability acknowledge the need to encourage active partnership with parents. There are growing efforts to demystify professional roles and to help parents use services more flexibly and in a more personalized way. Most health authorities now provide child development or district handicap teams whereby assessment and coordination can be provided in a coordinated manner. Such teams are usually based within a hospital or child development center and include social workers, teachers, and various other professionals. Increasingly, teams include a representative from a voluntary organization to ensure that parents have ready access to the support network of the local community.

Given the importance of how and when families are informed about their child's impairment, increasing study has been done on how diagnosis and early information are provided. One study (Cunningham & Davis, 1988) found that nearly 60% of the parents of children with Down syndrome were dissatisfied with the way they received the diagnosis and early services; accordingly one program has reorganized its practices based upon detailed interviews with parents. Among the new practices are: 1) always presenting diagnosis to both parents together with ample time for discussion, 2) always arranging a follow-up visit for further questions, 3) providing information that is both realistic and positively framed, and 4) making referrals to sources of ongoing support, both professional and community-based. For parents of children whose disability is identified at a later date, a different set of support activities have been developed taking into account that the family may have already found the parenting role less satisfying and furthermore may feel that valuable time has been lost.

This and other studies and the work of the Family Fund have shown the importance of recognizing the normal problems of childrearing, exacerbated in the circumstance of families with children with disabilities, families with low incomes, single parents, or those who are isolated by cultural or language difference. Among all families, behavior difficulties seem to cause the greatest disruption to family life. Early support through home-based learning programs, such as the Portage Home-Based Early Education Program, can greatly relieve emotional stress.

The availability of a "named person" or "key worker" is seen as a key factor in creating a supportive environment for parental involvement and emotional support. A number of initiatives have taken place in this area, including implementing the concept of a parent adviser as a member of a district handicap team in the East End of London, where families from minority ethnic groups often find local services bewildering and inaccessible without an advocate and interpreter. The 1981 Education Act, discussed in Chapter 6, makes provision for a "named person" to support parents during the assessment process. Although not implemented on a wide scale, where it does exist this support has served parents well where services are complex and where otherwise the right to participate in decision-making would be diluted and distorted by the confusion and emotional trauma surrounding assessment and diagnosis.

Voluntary organizations, both local and national, are an under-utilized resource by the formal caregiving system in the UK. There is a high potential in the voluntary sector for a variety of roles, ranging from befriending and counseling to sharing social and leisure activities, providing practical help and information, and advocacy. The Southend scheme uses trained parents as parent counselors following the diagnosis of disability. The Camden Elfrida Rathbone Projects provide advocacy and support during the formal assessment process. A recent study of self-help groups in London found that parents who used such groups were more satisfied with local government services, felt themselves to be more competent, and had more positive expectations for their children.

THE UNITED STATES OF AMERICA

In the United States of America prior to the 1960s caregiving families could count on little emotional support other than that which was available informally. In increasing number, however, family members have joined together to offer mutual support, and professionals have begun to structure programs to enhance the emotional well-being of caregiving families.

Numerous parent- and consumer-run organizations exist in the United States whose purposes include the provision of emotional support to caregiving families. Some, like the Spina Bifida Association or the Association for Retarded Citizens (ARC), center on certain types of disabling conditions. Organizationally, these consist of a national headquarters, with state and/or local chapters providing direct services. Other organizations may embrace a smaller constituency and represent local efforts designed to meet the needs of individual families regardless of disability type. Whether large or small, these parent-run (or initiated) programs focus on providing information and support to families. They let families know that they are not alone, that there is a common thread of support available from others with similar concerns.

Beginning in the 1980s, there has been a growing impetus among these organizations to join together in coalition. By doing so, individual organizations can enhance their capacity to provide information or support to families, and to influence policy. For example, at the national level Project CHAIN seeks to unite parent and parent-professional groups across the country; the National Institute on Disability and Rehabilitation Research has funded the Beach Center on Families and Disability at the University of Kansas and is supporting a major national study by the Human Services Research Institute and United Cerebral Palsy (UCP) of various approaches to supporting families who care for a child with a disability at home; there are statewide clearinghouses of self-help mutual support groups in more than 20 states and a National Self-Help Clearinghouse at The Graduate School and University Center, The City University of New York.

In partnership with families, professionals have helped to establish numerous parent-centered mutual support groups across the country. These provide needed emotional support, as well as encouraging family members to become active participants in the habilitative process and teaching parents how to become effecting advocates. For example, the Parent Education Advocacy Training Center in Virginia specializes in familiarizing parents with what they can expect of their local school districts, providing instruction in how to participate effectively in the design of their children's individual education program

(IEP), and showing families how to pursue legal recourse if they are unsatisfied with the services their children are offered. The PEAK Parent Center in Colorado has paid special attention to developing materials and conducting training efforts to provide an integrated education for all children.

URUGUAY

In Uruguay there are no permanent or systematic services devoted to helping the family in the process of coping with and overcoming the stress of having a child with a disability and the stresses during the various transition periods in the life of the child. A few efforts are underway, largely limited to voluntary groups addressing the needs of children with a particular type of disability and their families, for example, the parent associations that are members of PLENADI (National Federation of Disabled Persons). The Parents Training Center in Tarariras has developed a "From Family to Family Program," which incorporates "model parents" as primary agents of emotional support. These are parents whose child with a disability is older and, on this basis, it is believed that these parents are able to provide insight and support to parents of younger children.

CONCLUSION

Diversity among the nine countries in providing emotional support to families with a child with a disability ranges across not only the services provided, but also definition and purpose of services. This is seen particularly in the extent to which the need for emotional support is viewed as unique to families with a child with a disability. Another area of variability concerns the extent to which the focus is on provision of professional services versus the use of lay support, particularly mutual support from other families in a similar situation.

REFERENCES

Cunningham, C., & Davis, H. (1988). *Working with parents: Frameworks for collaboration.* London: Open University Press.

9

Employment, Housing, and Recreation

The focus of this book is on children with disabilities. Thus, attention to the issues of this chapter—employment, housing, and recreation—is not a matter of presenting extensive details about these areas in each of the nine countries. Rather, it is to sketch out the circumstances in each of them as a way to provide perspective in terms of the lives ahead of children with disabilities and their families.

AUSTRALIA

In Australia the provision of employment services rests primarily with the federal government either through funding of nongovernment agencies or through its rehabilitation service. The Disability Services Act of 1986 makes provision for two types of employment services: 1) supported employment and 2) competitive employment, training, and placement. Key features of the former are ongoing support to maintain and retain paid employment, valued work, working conditions similar to those in the general workforce, and integration with non-disabled persons in the work setting. Key features of the competitive employment services include wages and benefits consistent with those of nondisabled workers and integration with nondisabled persons in the work setting.

The act includes provision of a 5-year transition period for agencies running sheltered workshops and activity therapy centers to move to the new service designs. Some states are examining ways to provide better employment opportunities and move away from the day centers and activity programs which they currently conduct.

Overall, the states have a larger responsibility than the federal government for residential services, although a significant amount of federal government funding is provided to the private sector for these purposes. Some state housing departments are taking a greater interest in the provision of housing. For example, New South Wales and Western Australia have disability housing policies and in New South Wales there is a Disability Housing Unit.

The Federal Disability Services Act of 1986 includes accommodation support services as a service type, with the definition of assisting persons with disabilities to develop or maintain suitable residential arrangements in the community. The strategy under the act calls for agencies running larger hostels and nursing homes to change to smaller, more individualized accommodation support services.

Recreation and leisure activities are incorporated within the services covered by the Disability Services Act. These are to be freely selected from among a range of choices, be primarily for the purposes of personal satisfaction and enjoyment, contribute to the individual's well-being, and be age appropriate.

CANADA

In Canada, as noted in earlier chapters, there is an increasing emphasis on understanding services as part of the resources necessary to enable a family with a child with a disability to dream of a future and to make that dream into reality. This ability to dream is important to individuals and families throughout their lives. It is especially important at various points of transition in the life of the child, for example, when entering school, leaving school, entering adult life, and when the family is no longer available. To date, the responsiveness of the formal human services systems has been increasing inversely with the age of the individual; that is, the younger the individual the better the transition planning.

In various communities, however, creative activities are underway related to supported employment and supported community living. In both contexts, the focus has been on individual solutions and approaches, thus allowing the individual and the family to plan for the future. In addition, support circles are being developed that not only support successful transitions but also build quality lives. Associations for Community Living and similar groups are assisting families to develop options. In some communities, families have pooled resources available to them individually to develop services—both employment and recreational—that meet the needs of many children. A growing number of agencies are beginning to use transition points as the contexts for talking with families about the future, encouraging them to dream, and then organizing agency services to better assist in addressing the needs represented in those dreams.

ISRAEL

In Israel rehabilitation services aimed at providing gainful employment for persons with disabilities are provided by a number of agencies. The largest of these is the Rehabilitation Services Administration of the Ministry of Labor and Welfare. Its aim is to bring persons with handicaps to maximum nondependence upon the social service system and to place the person in an integrated work setting where she or he can earn a fair wage.

Where placement in such a setting is not possible because of the nature or extent or the handicap, employment in a sheltered setting is offered. Primarily, this is done through the Foundation of Rehabilitation Enterprises. Operating nationwide, the foundation's services include 15 rehabilitation centers, six long-term employment enterprises, two vocational centers for young persons, and three sheltered workshops for persons with a visual disability. The Department of Services for the Retarded operates 40 sheltered workshops for persons with mental disabilities. Additionally, sheltered workshops for persons with severe disabilities are provided by some voluntary organizations.

In keeping with the normalization principle, many services have set up hostels and shared housing units for persons with disabilities. For example, the Department of Services for the Retarded has 40 such living units in different parts of the country. There are also halfway houses for discharged psychiatric patients.

Social and recreational activities are provided by various agencies by category of disability. The Service for the Retarded has 35 social clubs for persons with a mental handicap dispersed throughout the country. These clubs provide supervised leisure time activities. Similar clubs provide services for persons with other impairments. For example, the Services for the Blind operates eight social clubs; ENOSH, a parent organization, has set up a number of social clubs for persons with psychiatric problems; NITZAN has clubs for youth with learning disabilities; ILAN has set up sports facilities; the Department of Rehabilitation, together with veterans groups, has built two sports and recreation centers for disabled veterans and their families; and the Organization for the Deaf has set up a dance group of both deaf and hearing dancers.

JAPAN

In Japan opportunities for persons with disabilities for gainful employment remain largely limited. There are, however, increasing opportunities for both sheltered employment and employment in a competitive setting. The Law for Promoting Employment of the Disabled stipulates that private businesses as well as government agencies are required to employ a certain number of persons with disabilities; until an amendment included persons with mental retardation, this covered only persons with physical disabilities. Organizations that do not meet this requirement are penalized, while those that exceed it receive a financial subsidy.

Vocational training is provided only to a limited extent in the schools. This is supplemented by training and vocational rehabilitation centers and on-the-job training, with the Public Employment Security Offices providing vocational placement and follow-up services.

Large sheltered workshops are operated by the government, while various private organizations and parent groups operate "mini-sheltered workshops." Many of these have less of an employment focus and serve more as a place for activities.

A new development is the work development centers for persons with mental retardation and severe physical disabilities. These are operated jointly by the public sector and a private company and provide prevocational and vocational training in a real work situation, with the goal being for the individuals to move into competitive employment.

The Welfare Laws for the Physically Disabled and for the Mentally Retarded provide group homes in the community, for 10–20 persons each. Some residential institutions that had been large are establishing smaller units, and there are smaller group homes that serve two or three persons in a family-like setting. Public subsidies are available for the physical adaptation of private homes, although funds for attendant care are not provided.

In large cities there are special sports (especially swimming) and recreation centers for persons with disabilities and hotel-like facilities at which persons with disabilities and their families can stay for short periods of time.

KENYA

In Kenya the provision of employment services goes back to colonial times. Churches initiated training for persons with disabilities, particularly blind persons and then for those with other physical handicaps. The provision of these services has been taken over by the government, assisted by nongovernmental organizations (NGOs), with the continuing involvement of many of the churches.

A 1968 act established a division within the Ministry of Culture and Social Services to train persons with physical disabilities for self-employment. In the first 10 years of the program's operation, it trained over 1,000 persons with physical disabilities in trades such as tailoring, shoemaking, agriculture, carpentry, welding, and jewelry making, as well as traditional crafts. The services have been geared to the rural areas where the bulk of the population lives and where major economic development activities are underway. The NGOs and the churches also conduct adult vocational training programs, including training of telephone operators, in farming, and for secretarial work.

There are no formal residential facilities or services for people with disabilities in Kenya. Most persons with disabilities live with their families, less by design than by circumstance. The Civitan Foundation is seeking to develop residential services to assist persons with disabilities who have jobs but no place to live. These are modeled after the small homes for school-age children with handicaps operated by the Catholic Church throughout the country. These homes cater to children in groups no larger than 12 whose homes are too far away from the schools.

The Vocational Rehabilitation Division of the Ministry of Culture and Social Services operates a Sports Association for persons with physical handicaps with the goal of developing sports facilities and competitions for persons with disabilities throughout the country. The Kenya National Sports for the Mentally Handicapped operates a similar program. And the Very Special Arts operates arts and recreational programs for persons with any disabilities.

SWEDEN

In Sweden adults with disabilities have the right to work. Depending on the nature and extent of the impairment, persons with disabilities work in competitive settings with assistance, in sheltered workshops, and in day centers. While these arrangements have gained response from native Swedes, among immigrant families sheltered work is less acceptable.

In the area of recreation county councils organized district teams, working in collaboration with community authorities and the different associations for sports and culture, and have developed what are called study circles among persons with developmental disabilities. A key need here is the training of persons to lead such groups, with the goal that every person with a disability has a choice of recreational opportunities that suit his or her interests and capacity.

There are no special housing provisions in Sweden for persons with disabilities.

THE UNITED KINGDOM

In the United Kingdom many day centers provide some form of assessment and preparation for work. And a number of Local Authorities now provide specialist employment agencies that help people find and keep jobs in the community. The Disablement Rehabilitation Officer also provides local advice and assistance. One particularly successful program is MENCAP's Pathway scheme, which supports people with mental handicaps during their first weeks on a new job and negotiates with the employer over any difficulties encountered. And some persons with disabilities are using a range of Training Commission (TC) schemes. The TC funds a major proportion of sheltered employment settings and is responsible for ensuring that young people with special needs have rights of access to a range of government-sponsored training programs.

The gradual closure of the long-stay mental handicap hospitals has laid the responsibility for provision of residential services on Local Authority social services departments. During the 1980s, the thrust toward care in the community has led to a number of important initiatives in enabling persons with disabilities to live in ordinary homes in their local communities, with necessary supports. This housing is often provided through local housing associations and increasingly through Local Authority housing departments. A number of voluntary organizations such as Barnardos and MENCAP and the village communities such as Home Farm Trust also provide a range of ordinary housing options.

Leisure activities are better developed for young children than for young adults. Some voluntary organizations such as MENCAP provide separate programs. However, there is increasing attention to encouraging young people with disabilities to participate in integrated local leisure activities.

THE UNITED STATES OF AMERICA

In the United States of America in 1984 the Assistant Secretary for Special Education and Rehabilitation Services, responding to the continued high rate of joblessness among adults with disabilities and the growing wave of youth who were "aging out" of their PL 94-142 entitlement, established a national priority on improving the transition from school to work life. The concept of transition was understood to encompass the latter years of schooling, as well as the initial years after graduation. Transitional programs have been developed throughout the country and usually include a functional, community-based curriculum; work experiences during the school years; collaboration with service providers for adults and with parents; and an individualized transition plan that encompasses vocational, residential, financial, social, and recreational goals.

Another major initiative established in the past several years to strengthen employment opportunities for persons with disabilities is supported employment. Until the 1980s, sheltered workshops were virtually the only employment option for persons with disabilities who were not able to perform independently at competitive rates. Supported employment involves paid work in an integrated setting. It encompasses job development and placement, intensive training at the job site, ongoing assessment, and provision of services essential to success at work. Many individuals with severe disabilities who were previously thought to be incapable of working or capable only of participating in sheltered work programs have now been able to demonstrate their ability to maintain employment in competitive work settings when provided with appropriate ongoing support.

While lack of opportunity, as well as outright discrimination, have been the strongest factors in keeping adults with disabilities out of paid competitive employment, another significant factor has been a disincentive, that is, the reduction of various public benefits or access to public programs. First on a trial basis and now as a permanent part of the Social Security system, many of these disincentives have been reduced or eliminated. Nonetheless, some disincentives, as well as lingering concern about the reality of the new changes, remain.

A part of a general employment strategy, the Targeted Jobs Tax Credit (TJTC) program has helped some adults with disabilities. TJTC provides subsidies to employers for the first months of the employment of persons with disabilities.

Since the mid-1970s there has been a dramatic shift from institutional to community living. Deinstitutionalization and integration into the community have been encompassed in the

Developmental Disabilities Act Amendments since 1975. Despite this, federal Medicaid dollars still go largely to support large public institutions. In the 1980s changing this situation has been the focus of concern, both nationally and in a number of states.

A key component of the effort to help persons with disabilities achieve greater independence is the network of more than 150 Centers for Independent Living (CIL) throughout the country, largely funded through federal rehabilitation legislation. The principles critical to the CILs are consumer involvement and control. CILs and independent living programs assist individuals with disabilities in all aspects of life in the community that are relevant to the achievement of greater independence. Personal assistance, as provided by attendants who help with routine activities of daily living, is one of the foci of many centers.

In the United States various structured recreational alternatives are available to persons with disabilities. In numerous communities, Special Olympics and other sports programs are offered. There are vacation camps for children with particular disabilities and some programs operated by self-advocacy groups such as People First.

While there are many programs, overall there is an absence of a comprehensive system of recreational opportunities for persons with disabilities. There is a growing consensus that recreational opportunities for persons with disabilities should not be established separate from those for persons who do not have disabilities. Thus, efforts are underway to utilize existing community structures (e.g., the Boy Scouts and Girl Scouts, the YWCA and YMCA, and Little Leagues) for the benefit of all, including persons with disabilities. And in some communities, youth service and recreational programs (e.g., the Alliance for Mainstreaming Youth with Disabilities) are coming together to advocate for and promote integrated activities.

URUGUAY

In Uruguay the government is legally obligated to employ persons with disabilities as up to 2% of the staff. However, high levels of unemployment and budget constraints have limited the enforcement of this provision.

Vocational programs for persons with disabilities were begun in the 1960s. Operating in schools and vocational workshops, they provide training programs for competitive work and preparation for Uruguay's very few sheltered workshops. Beginning in 1988, students with disabilities were integrated into the regular courses in all technical schools.

Out of home residential placements run contrary to the nation's strong commitment to family life and are very rare.

The Uruguayan Committee for Sports and Recreation of Disabled Persons (CUDEDI) is composed of private and public institutions working in the area of disability and sports and recreation. It includes the Committee for Special Olympics. Among CUDEDI's activities are training physical education teachers, training parents and community members to work with persons with disabilities in sports and recreational activities, and integrating persons with disabilities into general clubs and sports or recreation associations.

CONCLUSION

In all nine countries, opportunities for adults with disabilities to work and live in the community are limited; however, since the 1980s, employment and community living, and recreational opportunities as well, have grown, both overall, and as part of efforts to increase integration opportunities. While this has been the case in each of the nine countries, in none of them is the status of persons with disabilities equivalent to that of persons who do not have disabilities. This serves to limit the future opportunities for children with disabilities, and to increase the strains upon the families that seek to nurture them.

10

Conclusion

In responding to disability primary attention must be given to the preservation of the normal processes of human development, and the family and the community are the most important instruments for the working of those processes. (Acton, 1988, p. 5)

COMMUNITY AND CULTURAL CONTEXTS

While Acton, former Secretary General of World Rehabilitation, was writing in the context of nonindustrial countries, his point above has general meaning. So too, does his observation on community-based rehabilitation, echoing Goodman's (1989) point, which began Chapter 1, that attitudes and approaches come about (or are discouraged) through government policies. Werner (1988) takes the point a step further.

It [community-based rehabilitation] can be an extension of society's present demeaning, conciliatory, restrictive attitude toward the disabled, in which the goals of rehabilitation are too often to "train" and "normalize" the disabled to better fit into present social structure, however alienating and unjust this may be.

Or, it can be part of a grassroots struggle to transform society-at-large so as to provide more equal rights, respect, and opportunities for all who happen to be different, weaker [sic], disadvantaged. (p. 5)

Community-based rehabilitation does indeed involve a process of transformation. The traditional model assumes that persons with disabilities are "broken" and must be "fixed," with a concomitant assumption that society is right and needs no changing. Serpell (1988) points out that, instead, community rehabilitation is a process of mutual adaptation, which at its heart, recognizes that

> a society which seeks to empower its disabled members to achieve . . . the goal [of full participation by disabled individuals in the life of the society] thereby affirms its commitment to certain humane values. Only if the local community in which an individual lives accepts a significant degree of moral responsibility can the requisite process of mutual adaptation between society and individual take place. (p. 5)

Callahan (1988) offers a unique slant on the question of moral responsibility, asking what the ethical limits of a family's responsibility to provide care really are. His call for not only improved support services but also a richer moral culture seems warranted.

Serpell (1988) addresses one of the underlying themes of this book; namely, the cultural understanding of disability seen in the context of the extent to which practices in one type of country (those with advanced industrialized economies and social welfare systems) can be transferred to nonindustrial countries:

> The current pattern of professional rehabilitation practiced in the rich, industrialised countries of the West are an amalgam of technical responses to functional needs created by biological impairment and culturally specific forms of adaptation. Certain aspects of these practices can be transplanted to quite different societies without any loss of relevance, e.g., surgical interventions to correct a club foot or to remove a cataract. Moreover, this type of intervention can be implemented by a relatively small team of experts with minimal involvement of the community. Dramatic though the impact of these miracles of modern science has been, they are a dangerously atypical model of service developments as a whole.
>
> Other practices, such as the use of sign language, Braille printing, physiotherapy or behaviour modification have much wider social ramifications. The success or failure of these more representative techniques depends critically on direct family and community support over a period of months or years. A community which is struggling to survive in conditions of great economic

adversity will only incorporate such techniques within its existing cultural pattern of response to disability if they are clearly well
adapted to locally recognizable, priority needs. (p. 5)

Furthermore, in terms of community, Miles (1988) writes:

The bulk of desired assistance for people with disabilities has
been given, is now given, and probably will always be given, by
disabled people themselves, by families, friends, neighbours and
casual passers-by, regardless of any plan from New York or Pesh-
war, and without benefit of "expert validation." (p. 6)

These individuals from the community draw their responses from cultural, societal, and governmental contexts. In
a unique statement of governmental support, then-Prime Minister R.J.L. Hawke introduced a powerful official document,
Disability, Society and Social Change (1988), incorporating a
set of principles and derivative objectives for Australian society
that have been incorporated into the Disabilities Services Act of
1986. (See the Appendix to this chapter for excerpts from the
document.)

Werner (1988) notes the role that governments can play as
persons with disabilities become the subjects rather than the
objects in a truly empowering process:

Perhaps Sweden provides a useful model. When a recognized organization of disabled persons decides to promote or help sponsor
a particular program or initiative for and by disabled persons (in
Sweden or in a developing country), and when the organization of
disabled persons raises one-tenth of the funds needed, the Swedish government provides the remaining nine-tenths. In this way,
the collective of disabled persons has primary decision making
and control, while government and professional input is substantial but non-controlling. (p. 5)

However useful this Swedish model may be, we recognize that
aside from those technical interventions mentioned by Serpell
above, practices cannot be transferred intact from one country
or one cultural setting to another. Indeed, we are less sanguine
than Serpell even as to the ease of technical intervention trans-
fers, especially given the cultural meaning of particular disabling conditions. Nonetheless, we believe there are benefits in
looking at certain interventions within one country for their
possible meaning—not necessarily adaptation or adoption—in
other countries.

THE NINE COUNTRIES

It was this belief that led us to convene "A Cross-Cultural Conference for Families with a Child with a Disability," and to write this book. In Chapters 4 through 9 we have addressed various factors involved in support for families with a child with a disability in the nine countries represented at the conference. In the following section we present some of the special insights of the team members representing each of the nine countries. While the countries and their activities vary widely, it is apposite to note that among them are some common themes, including a growing understanding of disability as a social construct, the need to recognize the family consequences of having a member with a disability, the importance of recognizing both the varied cultural understandings of and response to disability, and the context of the country's social welfare system.

Australia

The Australian team identified the following issues for particular attention:

> The influence of geography on service delivery. This may, for example, lead to considerable discrepancy in quality and quantity of services across a given region or area. This creates equity and access problems.
>
> A multi-cultural society faces particular problems in information dissemination and service delivery because of customs, language and cultural factors.
>
> Parents of a child with a disability should have access to relevant information at the appropriate time on a range of matters, including facts on the child's short and long term prognosis, location of services, supports, assistance, etc. Information difficulties, such as delays and misinformation, can have a considerable negative impact on the family, resulting in unnecessary stress and lost opportunities. People who have immediate contact with new parents are frequently the least informed about these matters.
>
> Integration and/or linking of services and service information is very important. This includes social security arrangements that form an integrated system of financial support for families and young people with disabilities. This principle recognizes the overlap or potential overlap and interaction between cash benefits, education grants, training allowances, service and other forms of support for families and young people. The aim would be to increase consistency and equity between different arrangements and programs and States/Territories within a country.

Family supports, including income supports, should recognize the growing independence of young people with disabilities. This suggests that increased independence (including financial) is an important factor in the attainment of adult status regardless of the disability of the young person.

While research, development and demonstration activities are a vital part of any dynamic human service system, there is frequently a gap between what is achievable during these activities and what occurs generally in service delivery. The gap can sometimes be very large. Innovative methods need to be used to ensure that research and development findings are translated into general practice.

A key requirement for priority setting, planning, service delivery and research is the endorsement by a broad range of interest groups, including governments, of clear philosophical statements which promote a valued place in society for people with a disability. (Ellis, Limbrick, Scibilia, & Sharpes, 1989, pp. 32–33.)

Canada

The Canadian team focused on natural settings, more creative policy, and consistency between policy rhetoric and implementation:

There are growing numbers of services which truly respond to the needs of families. There are increasing efforts to reshape and involve the community in the lives of families and people with handicaps. Families are being enabled to exercise power and decision making control. There is an increasing recognition of the handicapping nature of the social and physical environment.

We are also concerned about a number of dimensions of the Canadian reality which frustrate these trends:

Across Canada, we have examples of excellent responses to individual, family, and community needs. They are built on respect and responsiveness. Together they can help us see, in composite, what our vision of quality would begin to look like were all of the examples available in one community. At the same time, we are acutely aware of the fact that these examples are only examples. We do not have a community which has succeeded in creating a range of positive options. Some excel in different areas. Many provide a limiting array of traditional approaches. None excel in all areas.

Our vision of what is possible and desirable, based on the best that exists across the country, is expanding rapidly. Government and agency policies are increasingly, though far from systematically, coming into line with that vision. At the same time, the gap between the vision and the reality faced by families and individuals widens across Canada.

The gaps between government policy rhetoric and the reality of funding and implementation are often quite wide.

There is a growing emphasis on seeing people with disabilities as people who have the same needs as everyone else. At the same time, there is a stubborn tendency for services to see the needs of people in terms of a service. John is seen as needing a group home, rather than in need of a home, people to live with who are of his own choosing, neighbours who will grow to share his life, and so on. Families are seen to need counselling to deal with their frustrations, rather than support to overcome the obstacles which cause the frustrations.

Increasingly, government policy and funding are moving in the direction of supporting families and new approaches to ensure community presence, participation, and dignity. At the same time, new policy and funds are often only add-ons to the existing situation. Restrictive, non-supportive services are maintained, while approaches which support and build on inclusion and involvement are permitted. Rarely does policy place the priority on the development of responsive options. Rarely are agencies compelled or offered incentives to move in more creative directions. (Kappel, Lusthaus, & Snow, 1989, pp. 36–37)

Israel

The focus in Israel is on professional services, here made more complex by the intertwining of public and private providers:

1. Most of the systems and services are provided by government departments.
2. The government maintains these systems and provides these services by means of a large number of agencies.
3. These branches deliver services directly to their clients through local branches that operate either independently or in cooperation with local government.
4. No formal network for the coordination of these agencies' activities exists. As a result of this, there is a fragmentation of services, many of these services are sporadic, and there is no clear national policy or guidelines for determining need and initiation of services.
5. Families in urban areas have better services than families in rural areas.
6. Although Arab citizens have the same rights, their utilization of services are [sic] not equal and this population should be helped to improve their consumerism.
7. There is no guideline for division of services according to type of disability or type of services. Often the same service exists for all disability types without distinction of special needs.

8. Due to budgetary limitations and the reduction in public services, private support services for families have become more common and families are beginning to avail themselves of these services. This may create some inequality in obtaining services for low-income families.

9. Family support services usually have an individual focus. The State allows a family of a child with a disability to buy a vehicle without taxes, but little is done at a national level to make public transportation accessible to all persons with a handicap. A similar situation exists in housing. If new buildings are standardly made accessible, then there would not be the need for special services for renovations.

10. There is a need for specific parent support services in the area of transition. This is a particularly important area of concern, which in Israel has not received adequate attention. Parents need help in planning their children's transition from school to further education or work, transition from institution or foster care to community, and transition from family home to independent living.

11. Social support services for helping families contribute to the independent living of their children with disabilities are still in their infancy. Parents have a social mandate to be mentors of their children, especially with regard to the sensitive area of interpersonal and sexual behavior. Parents require considerably more professional support in fulfilling this mandate, especially in the attainment of skills and emotional insight into the problems related to the sexuality of their children and to independent living. (Florian & Katz, 1989, pp. 24–26)

Japan

In Japan, services for persons with disabilities are rapidly emerging:

Services for the disabled in Japan have been greatly developed for the last 10 years or so. Various techniques for early intervention have been developed. . . . It has been widely accepted that disabled children are helped in the full development of their full potential when they are integrated in a group of normal children and given as many opportunities as possible for learning and socialization.

Integration into ordinary schools has not been so pervasive. The Ministry of Education never uses the word "integration". At the local level, some local authorities have a more positive attitude toward "integration". When we consider segregation in schools in regard to the education of disabled children, we cannot overlook the reality that schools have been busy producing candidates for a labor force that has contributed to Japan's high rate of economic development. The same can be said about the situation for adults with disabilities in seeking to achieve independence in the general society of Japan.

The International Year of Disabled Persons has been an epoch-making activity, in which the issue of social independence of disabled persons has received serious attention from the society in general for the first time in Japan. However, we still hear parents say, "When I die, I cannot leave my disabled child behind." These words symbolize that services for the disabled are still not sufficient to ensure a quality of life for them. It is also a reflection of the idea in our culture that the child is a part of its parents' belongings without recognizing the child as an independent person.

It is true that in today's Japan wider varieties of services for the disabled are available. It, however, is not yet enough. Most of the parents of disabled children have the experience of doctor shopping and running around from one agency to another in order to find appropriate information regarding available services for their disabled child. Lack of coordination of services has long been a big problem, yet to be solved. The coordination needs to be horizontal between related offices and agencies as well as vertical between higher levels of administration and more local ones. . . . Disabled children and their families are often left out without receiving appropriate services between cracks in the system.

Rapid industrialization and urbanization has necessarily resulted in a change in family systems, a change from an extended family to a nuclear family. On account of this change, some family functions need to be transferred outside of the family. Home help services are far from enough to meet needs both in quantity and quality. More flexibility in service hours and more varieties of services are required in order to meet the complex needs of families with disabled children. Respite care is another type of care service that is badly needed. In our culture, leisure time activities have been valued rather low in one's life, with higher value being placed upon hard work. Parents tend to be afraid of criticism from others if they take a break leaving their disabled children under some other's care even briefly. The idea, however, has been gradually accepted that taking a break has vital meaning in order to enable parents to regain energy to provide a better family environment for all members of the family, including the disabled child.

In Japan, it is quite common for young adults before their marriage to live with their parents. Normally, they leave their parents' home when they get married, but sometimes young couples live with parents after their marriage. . . . It has been customary that parents would keep their grown up disabled child at home. Today, however, not only physically disabled persons but also mentally retarded persons are seeking community living. The situation is hard for the severely disabled. They are often forced to stay home without any day programs for them to participate in their community. There are many mini-sheltered workshops throughout the country, to which the national government and local authorities give certain subsidies. One of the problems with this type of program is that the subsidies are too small to employ enough staff, and parents, especially mothers, must work side-by-side with their grown children all day. This is not really a form of integration.

In this aging society, issues surrounding care of the disabled are not merely the problems to be solved for the disabled. There are cases in which the aged disabled are taking care of their elderly parents. Support services for families with disabled adults are still to be developed.

In order to actualize the philosophy of "normalization", a wide range of community-based services have to be provided. Those which are already in existence need to be improved, and many more services have to be developed. In Japan, community-based services for promoting integration of disabled persons are still rather new. Community-based services should be comprehensive and designed in such a way as to effectively meet the needs of disabled persons and their families in their community. (Oi, Higuchi, & Takei, 1989, pp. 28–30)

Kenya

Kenya has the most limited resources of all the nine countries:

> Support systems for families with disabled children have not been developed in the country. This seems to have come about, first, because of the cultural and traditional outlook of the people and second, the stage of development of services for disabled persons.
>
> Lack of financial assistance and personnel has contributed negatively to the provision of services to disabled persons and their families. This situation will continue for quite a long time to come as long as training services in the country are still lacking in many areas, especially in disability. Coupled with this are the two problems of communication and ignorance among families with disabled children. Attempts by parent organizations such as the Civitan Foundation and others to address the issue will have less of an impact because of constraints related to finances and personnel. Other attempts by the government will also meet with the same constraints.
>
> [I]mprovement of services to families with disabled persons is a route that developing countries will have to pursue vigorously. Such assistance should be in the form of developing local capabilities to deal with local problems.
>
> [F]inally, the development and implementation of family support services in developing countries like Kenya should incorporate local traditional aspects so that the noble cultural practices are continued and perfected. Such an approach will enrich the

culture and promote better appreciation of the tribal differences among the different ethnic groups in the country. (Odeck, 1989, pp. 33–34)

Sweden

Sweden has an advanced social welfare system. Complications arise, however, as these services are extended to immigrant groups:

People's attitudes toward disability can be explained by many different causes. One of them has to do with the socio-economic development in the country. A country with good economic development can permit itself to be generous toward minority groups, including immigrants and disabled persons. For Sweden, this has involved immigrants from Yugoslavia, Greece and Turkey. The institutions built to give care and education for disabled children are more in response to the state's possibilities than to the needs of the disabled children and their families.

On the individual level, immigrant parents do not accept the help they may need. This is a result of several difficulties in combination. There is the maladjustment to the life in the new society with homesickness and idealizing of life in the old country. The arrival of a disabled child increases the stress. Often, the emotional conflict is denied. The parents try to cope with the situation, the women with isolation and the men with flight. As they deny their feelings of harm and sorrow, they have few possibilities to understand the information given about their child. They may react to the conflict by developing psychosomatic disorders. If the disabled child is born in Sweden, the parents may have magic thoughts that it will be healed going back to the home country. Only when the parents, often after years of struggle, have accepted the condition can they do something about it. They can accept help and ask for services. They start to collaborate with different experts around the needs of their child. When the immigrant parents accept the whole situation they start to be interested in treatment and care offered by Swedish services. Before they waited for a miracle and tried all sorts of cures. Parents sacrifice in effort, time and money as if it were possible to turn the cruel fate into fortune. The success may not be in healing the child's disability but in a reevaluation of what is important in life. The reevaluation may even open their minds to accept that they need help, help to express their denied feelings and reach their original strength again.

The well-organized society in Sweden is often incomprehensible to immigrant families. Misunderstandings are frequent, although interpreters are engaged to help the immigrants with their contacts with official services.

Oral information to a group of parents with the same cultural background is the most efficient method to inform them about services, regulations, treatments, training and education. Immigrant parents with disabled children often are isolated. Through programs of parent education, parents come together, get useful information and knowledge at the same time as they make friends. They share experiences and they give each other emotional support. They recognize that they are not alone in a hopeless situation. They can even compare themselves with Swedish families with disabled children. Many experiences and feelings are common and the need for support exists in all groups. It is the way to search for it, to show the need of support, and the way to solve problems that are different from one cultural group to another. (Riden, Wastberg, & Wendelholt, 1988, pp. 12–14)

The United Kingdom

In the United Kingdom changes in services for persons with disabilities and their families are occurring as broader public policies intersect with social developments. Particular attention is being given to ways to encourage professional services to support families' autonomy and enhance their capacity:

Genuine partnership with parents necessitates a relationship in which the professional services work *with* [italics in the original] parents by making appropriate expertise available to them. The relationship is, therefore, one of complementary expertise, since the expert knowledge of the parents of themselves, their aims, their situation, their child complements what the professionals can offer. Good services for children—involving negotiated individual programmes and agreed collaborative procedures between professionals—will not only maximize the child's development but establish important principles for subsequent services for adults. Recent evaluations of users' satisfaction with early intervention services clearly demonstrates that early and flexible intervention does produce more positive attitudes in parents; does appear to enable parents to keep severely handicapped children at home and can benefit the individual child's development. Furthermore, it offers accessible resources to the wide range of professionals within child health services, social services and education who are concerned in providing services to meet the needs of handicapped children and their families. However, early intervention is ineffective without a continuing and comprehensive range of support services reflecting changing individual needs.

Parents clearly gain from mutual support and friendship. Health and Education authorities and social services departments should ensure that parents are aware of local self-help and voluntary networks which can offer advice, counselling and practical support. Parent groups and voluntary organizations have an additional role in providing consultative groups for the development of local services and as part of an evaluative process in assessing the effectiveness and appropriateness of current service provision.

A centre or team can act as a base of effective referral of families to neighbourhood community services. Many parents criticize the fragmentation and duplication of services. The team approach avoids such duplication and or waste and (with the use of a key worker or named person) ensures that parents are aware of options for help and are able to make use of them.

Definitions of "family" need to be construed widely, since many children will increasingly live in substitute families or in small group homes in the community. Foster parents or staff acting "in loco parentis" in the community should have access to *parent* [italics in the original] services.

Many families need a flexible service to cover particular needs. Provision for flexibility necessitates particular attention to patterns of referral and use; to consumer and professional evaluation and to a team approach in order to ensure that families are neither isolated and forgotten or subject to "over-kill" from competing professionals. Services for children should not only focus on *early* [italics in the original] intervention, but develop a lifecycle and incremental approach with particular reference to periods of transition such as transfer to full-time school or to adult services. Key professionals working with families should have a knowledge of *normal* [italics in the original] child development and child-care, as well as a capacity to cope with specific difficulties relating to the mental handicap. Integration should be seen as planned interaction in *all* [italics in the original] aspects of daily life.

Family support cannot flourish without effective management and sufficient resources. The Griffiths Report on Community Care stressed the major implications for future patterns of services of the growth of a mixed economy of provision. The growing number of private and voluntary residential services highlights the need for central government to take community care very seriously. Without some strategic central overview, services for disabled people may become fragmented and isolated. In a mixed economy of welfare services, social services may find themselves less frequently providers and more often social care agents. Case management will be crucial, since there will be a multiplicity of provision of variable quality. There are genuine fears that people with complex disabilities or challenging behaviours might not be acceptable to the new market forces in community care without more effective targeting of resources. . . . In the last resort parents and disabled people are likely to be the strong and committed "champions of change". But they will have a voice only if central and local government are willing to make consumer involvement in choice and quality control a major priority. (Mittler & Russell, 1989, pp. 51–54)

The United States of America

In the United States of America there is both growing provision of professional services and increasing recognition of the importance of community and informal resources. The ways these two relate, in a time both of growing assertion of disability rights and increasing diversity in the forms and functions of families, is a central development:

> For policy makers, establishing means for strengthening the family fabric within American society must be a foremost concern. Key to their success will be an underlying respect for the differences among families, including those distinctions based in culture and custom. Moreover, policy makers must not overlook the growing need for a coherent national policy directed at assuring that all families will have access to needed supports.
>
> In this regard, families would benefit, first of all, from policies that are directed toward strengthening families in general. Given the population dynamics, . . . there is need for a great variety of family centered programs to: 1. reduce teenage parenthood, 2. assure every family with children an income at least at the poverty line, 3. assure adequate housing for families with low income, 4. assure adequate health care for all, including those with disabilities, 5. provide maternity and paternity leave with benefits for parents of a young infant, 6. assure the availability of suitable child care for working parents, and 7. provide greater flexibility in work hours for parents.
>
> [F]amilies who provide care at home to children with disabilities also deserve a system that supports them in accordance with their individual, unique patterns of needs and strengths; a system that is comprehensive and coordinated; a system that recognizes the financial strain that many low and middle income families experience in caring for children with severe disabilities at home, and that provides ways to ease this strain; a system that is equitable to families irrespective of the part of the United States in which they reside; a system that enables them to pursue normative patterns of living.
>
> [F]amily support programs will not reach all those in need in ways consistent with the emerging goals and themes presented above unless two processes take place: 1. families organize and advocate effectively on their own behalf, and 2. professionals perceive and define themselves not only as service providers but also as partners with families in advocating for systemic change. The challenge facing family members and professionals is to forge

such a partnership and use it to shape public policy. (Cohen, Agosta, Cohen, & Warren, 1989, pp. 43–44)

Uruguay

In a sense, Uruguay is a country in the middle, advanced in concepts of issues of disability and family support, yet facing severe financial constraints:

> The current situation is, in general terms but with a few exceptions, one of divergence between conceptual beliefs and reality of services at the operational level. The prospects for improvement of this ambivalent situation are very positive, since changes at all levels are observed: at the government level [where] Congress is considering three laws on disability . . . ; at the professional level [where there is] growing acceptance of the interdisciplinary approach . . . ; at the level of disabled persons and of the responsible organizations [where there is] awareness and group action leading to accepting the need for an integrative approach since all community components are interdependent and contrary to the situation of two decades ago, it is more than ever evident that the participation of the disabled persons and their families in the planning, operation and decision-making is important; at the community level [where] a weak response is visible that has moved from a deep rejection of the disabled person to an implicit acceptance, which provides an indicator of an attitudinal change in process; and at the family level.

> It is recommended
> That provisions for the protection and integration of the disabled person/family and family/community units be included in national legislation.
> That strategies be designed so that social security, health and education services function in a systematic integrated approach to the family of the disabled, and not only focussed upon the disabled individual.
> That census items be included in the National Census or specific surveys which permit quantification of disability factors.
> That research be conducted so as to define family structure, as well as to describe different types of families and factors affecting their dynamics.
> That the family of the disabled person be incorporated in the planning and the operational phases of the programs affecting them.
> That integration models be designed for the different types of support services to families of disabled persons, which should be planned with the habilitation and rehabilitation systems (at the local, regional and national levels) . . . .

That there be the creation and operation of parents' advocacy programs or support programs (for and of parents) as an essential service for the family, a concept and practice not quite developed in Latin America.

That in the training curriculum of professionals, specialists and community leaders incorporate content on disability and its prevention, the risk concept and the nature of habilitation and rehabilitation processes.

That there be information dissemination [that] stress[es] the importance of an international network of people and organizations involved in community integration of people with disabilities, [and that] stress[es] the importance of sharing information and experiences of developing support systems for the family, and the organization of international networks of people who are working towards the goal of community integration. (Speranza, 1989, pp. 33–38)

TOWARD A BROADER VISION OF FAMILY SUPPORT

Family support systems have been developed in many countries as a result of the recognition that the consequences of disability affect both the individual with disabilities and the other members of her or his family. Within the context of this understanding, the issue becomes the nature of the support to be provided, affected by the characteristics of the family and its dynamics and the individual with a disability and her or his characteristics.

As Lipsky (1985) points out, "stress is most often not a factor of psychological dysfunction but, rather, the absence of sympathetic social or economic systems" (p. 617). Also, McKaig (1986) notes that the situation facing the family is not solely internal.

> *Major sources of stress within families who care for their children at home are due more to external factors* [italics in the original] than to the responsibilities of parenting a child with demanding needs. Families repeatedly report social isolation, even ostracism and constant confrontations born of ignorance, stereotyped attitudes and prejudice. The difficulties of dealing with recalcitrant, fragmented and underdeveloped service networks takes an enormous physical and emotional toll on families. And, finally, the prospect of prolonged, unrelieved care-giving weighs heavily. (McKaig, 1986, p. 22)

The definition of "family support" varies widely in the different regions of the United States and in other countries. At its root, however, is the recognition that a family "offers stability, consistency and close relationships which cannot be duplicated. . . . Like other people, the quality of life for . . . disabled people is at its best when they can live in their home" (*Family support services*, 1986, p. 1).

In considering the establishment of family support services, Lipsky (1989) cautions that the following five factors need to be considered:

1. The dangers in most professional formulations of the consequences of disability for a family, which emphasize pathology and ascribe deviancy, necessitating professional treatment of any family response
2. The potential that in understanding the family consequences (i.e., the impact upon the nondisabled members), the special and unique needs of the individual with the disability will be downplayed if not ignored
3. The need to recognize that families differ, in composition, needs, cultural heritage, life stage, each of which affect their understanding of and reaction to disability
4. The need to address a set of gender issues—both the special issues involved for women with disabilities (Fine & Asch, 1988) and the special caregiver responsibilities that many cultures assign to women
5. The unique feature that unlike traditional minority families seeking to buffer and protect each other from the hostility of the larger society, the child with a disability is (most often) a member of a family which does not share in the experience (or culture) of disability. Thus, in addition to the strengthening that comes from a strong system of family supports, children with disabilities need opportunities to be with and learn from other persons with disabilities. (pp. 171–172)

Agosta (1989), who has conducted a number of studies of family support programs in the United States (cf. Agosta, Bass, & Spence, 1986; Agosta, Bradley, Rugg, Spence, & Covert, 1985; Agosta, Langer-Ellison, & Moore, 1988), emphasizes that, while all family support programs by definition are family-centered, what this means is not always entirely clear. He identifies three conceptual underpinnings: 1) services should enable and empower family members to make informed decisions; 2) services should be responsive to the needs of the entire family unit; and 3) services should be flexible enough to accommodate unique needs.

For services to enable and empower family members to make informed decisions, it is necessary to recognize that when family members "fail to display needed skills to do so [it is] not because of irreconcilable personal deficits, but instead [they] do so primarily due to an absence of sufficient opportunities to acquire needed competencies" (Agosta, 1989, p. 191). In recognition of this, Dunst (1986) recommends that families have enabling experiences wherein such competencies can be gained and displayed. Furthermore, for family members to lay "claim to control over their lives, . . . they must attribute the changes in their lives to their own actions" (Agosta, 1989, p. 191). Darling (1988) points out that parents often feel (in truth, often are made to feel) a sense of powerlessness, one of the components of anomie, when they see "their child's treatment as totally in the hands of professionals, thus obscuring their parental role" (cited in Agosta, 1989, p. 146).

In responding to the needs of the entire family unit, as Johnson (1979) emphasizes,

> the family is viewed as an interacting and reacting system that is delicately balanced and struggles to maintain that balance. A change or problem in one aspect of the system affects the entire system. (cited in Agosta, 1989, p. 192)

The need for flexibility in services grows from the reality that no two families, with or without children with disabilities, are alike. Considerable variation exists within families; moreover, families' needs evolve and change over time. A major factor in the variations between families concerns culture:

> To be most effective, support services must be consistent with the culturally based preferences of individual families. This holds true regardless of the number of families sharing a particular belief system or the degree of difference between the dominant and minority cultures. (Agosta, 1989, p. 192)

Turnbull and Turnbull (1989) offer a contrast between "traditional" and "state-of-the-art" practices concerning family support. (See Table 10.1.)

As background for a project to promote family support programs, funded by the National Institute on Disability and Rehabilitation Research (HSRI/UCPA receive NIDRR grant on family support policy, 1986), United Cerebral Palsy of America identified the essential components of family support:

Table 10.1.   Family support services

Traditional	State of the art
1. Parents' greatest need (to which professional counseling and advice is geared) is to accept the burden of raising their child and to become realistic about his or her limitations and the fact that disability necessarily results in second-class citizenship.	1. Families need to be encouraged to dream about what they want for themselves and the person with a disability; and they need assistance in making those dreams come true. This assistance can include help in future planning. These dreams and future plans should lead to expectations that all members of the family are entitled to full citizenship. Planning to fulfill dreams should result in diminished needs for counseling, as empowerment through future planning replaces despair.
2. Parents' difficulties in coping with the child are largely psychological or psychiatric in nature, and the proper interventions are psychiatric or psychological counseling.	2. Families can benefit from each other. One benefit that almost all families need is the emotional resiliency and information that other families have acquired about life with disability. Thus, families need mentor programs that combine experienced and inexperienced families.
3. Mothers need respite to alleviate the stress and burden of caring for their child.	3. Families need for the person to have friends and integrated recreational options to respond to the person's needs for socialization, affection, and identity. Inter-personal relationships should supplement the caretaking model.

(continued)

Table 10.1.   (continued)

Traditional	State of the art
	Simultaneously, while the person is engaged in personalized and preferred activities, other family members will have opportunities to attend to their own needs. For some families, traditional respite care may still be necessary but it is rarely sufficient.
4. Mothers need clinical information about disability.	4. Families need information about and inspiration from people with a disability who are successfully integrated into community life. Clinical information, alone, does not inspire and raise expectations; indeed, it can do the opposite.
5. Mothers need training related to skill development and behavior management so they can be "follow-through" teachers for their child and implement home-based lesson plans.	5. Families need encouragement and ways to ensure that the person has a functional education taught in natural environments. This encouragement and help should assist families to enlist the support of the natural helpers in those environments (e.g., family, friends, store clerks, bus drivers, scout leaders). In this way, community-based education will contribute to further skill development and generalization. This means that families need some of the traditional

(continued)

Table 10.1.   (continued)

Traditional	State of the art
	clinical knowledge, too, but for different reasons and different outcomes.
6. Parents need training on how to advocate for the implementation of existing rights for their child.	6. Families need to know how to advocate, and obtain help in advocating for changes in service systems so that the systems will help satisfy the family's dreams for the person and the entire family.
7. Many families are financially unable to meet their child's needs and should seek out-of-home placement.	7. Many families need new policies to provide, for example, direct subsidies and new tax credits, to help meet the financial demands associated with disability in the home and family setting.
8. The child who poses unusual difficulties for a family should be separated from the family and placed in an institution or other congregate care setting.	8. Rather than the automatic assumption of out-of-home placement, families need to learn how to communicate among themselves about their dreams and the reality of family life. They need to know how to communicate among themselves about making those dreams come true, how to solve and prevent problems, and how to develop other capacities for community living and integrated services.
9. Parents of adults with disabilities have no support needs beyond learning how to "let go."	9. Families have a variety of support needs over the entire life span.

(continued)

Table 10.1. (continued)

Traditional	State of the art
10. White, middle-class, two-parent families are the family style of choice in this society; minority groups and nontraditional families should be provided with assistance to achieve that style.	10. Minority and nontraditional families may have strengths and support strategies that are as effective, or even more so, than white, middle-class families. Support should be developed to supplement individual family styles.

(Adapted from Turnbull & Turnbull [1989], pp. 11–13.)

the support in family support should be defined by the family
families need to be supported in defining their needs as well as
    have their needs met
the effectiveness of support services should be determined by
    their responsiveness in meeting the needs defined by the
    families
family support programs should respect that families are in con-
    trol and should trust that parents know what is needed
services should be delivered regardless of family income
services should not attempt to fit the person to the program
services should focus on the whole family—not just the family
    member with the disability
parents should be given time to build trust
parents experience life passages and will need different support
    and/or services at different points
professionals need to be sensitive about and to families—families
    can be used to train professionals
families should have convenient and central access to "the sys-
    tem"
the natural supports in the community should be encouraged:
    relatives, neighbors, and friends
the system must be label-free and respond quickly
special equipment should be designed and built "to live in a
    family"
family support services should include options from an array of
    services, developed and chosen by families (Smith, 1987, p.4)

A local New York City program that works with low-income
and largely minority families whose children have significant
developmental disabilities, summarizes the following principles of service planning:

Services should *support* [italics in the original] not supplant, families.

Services should be provided in settings which are as typical and *integrated* [italics in the original] as possible into normal routines of life.

Services should offer *flexibility* [italics in the original].

Services should represent the complete *diversity* [italics in the original] of need.

Services should be provided on a *life-long* [italics in the original] basis.

Services should be offered with *competence* [italics in the original] based upon needs of the child and circumstances of the family. (McKaig, 1986, p. 38)

While it is premature to suggest a template for family support in the United States, or in the world as a whole, Lipsky (1987), having surveyed family support programs in several countries, presents a broad conception of the characteristics of an effective family support system:

early initiation, that is the system reaches out to the family at the beginning of the family's involvement;

integrated services, while families will begin with one or another need, most often there will be a variety of needs, generally meetable by differing agencies. Whatever the institutional reasons for this, from the family's perspective receipt of the array of needed services should not be a function of agency territorial lines or eligibility criteria or service plans or professional prerogatives;

a concomitant of this is **universal access,** that wherever a family enters the system, all parts should be available to them;

while the totality of services may run a wide range, for any individual family it is its **unique set of needs** that must be addressed—in effect selection from a **cafeteria of services**;

while we have talked of a family's needs, in fact the members of the family have unique needs, both the person with disabilities and the other individual members, so that the services must be **individualized**;

while supports are designed to respond to needs, they should be designed to **build upon and bolster strengths** and not focus on deficits;

the shared experiences of families with a disabled member offer the basis for **mutual support** among such families;

paramount recognition needs to be given to the family's capacity, including the ability to determine their own needs. Thus, in determination of needs and the ways to meet them, the wishes of the family and of its members should be given priority. (pp. 10–11)

This last point, the family's determination of its own needs, raises questions about the basic structure of family support programs. Programs with fixed components almost always prove to be of limited usefulness because they either squeeze the family's needs into a pre-established pattern or they fail to meet the full range of the family's needs. While not without complications, more for the bureaucracy however than for the families, cash assistance (Agosta, 1989) and voucher programs (McKaig, 1986) bear serious consideration.

EQUAL RIGHTS AND EQUAL OBLIGATIONS

Children with disabilities are neither rewards to nor punishments for their families, although at times, as with all children, they may seem like either or both. And, as with all children, they present both burden and opportunity to the family. They are entitled, as are all children, to be nurtured and loved, to hope and aspire, to have opportunities to contribute to society, to live in the community with family and friends.

Three principles from the United Nations World Programme of Action Covering Disabled Persons, adopted by the General Assembly in 1982, bear noting here:

25. The principle of equal rights for the disabled and the non-disabled implies that needs of each and every individual are of equal importance, that these needs must be made the basis for the planning of societies, and that all resources must be employed in such a way as to ensure, for each individual, equal opportunity for participation. Disability policies should ensure the access of the disabled to all community services.

26. As disabled persons have equal rights, they also have equal obligations. It is their duty to take part in the building of society. Societies must raise the level of expectation as far as disabled persons are concerned, and in so doing mobilize their full resources for social change.

27. Persons with disabilities should be expected to fulfill their role in society and meet their obligations as adults. The image of disabled persons depends on social attitudes based on different factors that may be the greatest barrier to participation and equality. (*World Programme*, 1983, p. 7)

Effective family support programs are essential for equal rights and equal opportunity for persons with disabilities.

REFERENCES

Acton, N. (1988). Community-based rehabilitation. *International Rehabilitation Review, 39* (2–3), 5.

Agosta, J. (1989). Using cash assistance to support family efforts. In G.H.S. Singer & L.K. Irvin (Eds.), *Support for caregiving families: Enabling positive adaptation to disability* (pp. 189–204). Baltimore: Paul H. Brookes Publishing Co.

Agosta, J.M., Bass, A., & Spence, R. (1986). *The needs of families: Results of a statewide survey in Massachusetts.* Cambridge, MA: Human Services Research Institute.

Agosta, J.M., Bradley, V.J., Rugg, A., Spence, R., & Covert, S. (1985). *Designing programs to support family care for persons with developmental disabilities: A growing commitment* (pp. 94–112). Cambridge, MA: Human Services Research Institute.

Agosta, J.M., Langer-Ellison, M., & Moore, K. (1988). *The feasibility of implementing a MDDPC sponsored cash assistance family support program.* Boston: Developmental Disabilities Planning Council.

Callahan, D. (1988). Families as caregivers: The limits of morality. *Archives of Physical Medicine and Rehabilitation, 69,* 13–18.

Cohen, S., Agosta, J., Cohen, J., & Warren, R. (1989). Supporting families with disabilities in the United States of America. In *Supports for families with a disabled child: Collected papers from an International Cross-Cultural Conference.* New York: The Graduate School and University Center, The City University of New York.

Disability, society and social change. (1988). Canberra, Australia: Commonwealth of Australia.

Dunst, C. (1986). *Helping relationships and enabling and empowering families.* Morgantown, NC: Family, Infant and Preschool Program, Western Carolina Center.

Ellis, J., Limbrick, D., Scibilia, S., & Sharpes, J. (1989). Australian services and programs to support families who have a child with a disability. In *Supports for families with a disabled child: Collected papers from an International Cross-Cultural Conference.* New York: The Graduate School and University Center, The City University of New York.

Family support services: Expanding alternatives for families with developmentally disabled individuals. (1986). Albany: Office of Mental Retardation and Developmental Disabilities.

Fine, M., & Asch, A. (1988). *Women with disabilities.* Philadelphia: Temple University Press.

Florian, V., & Katz, S. (1989). Support systems for a child who has a disability: An Israeli perspective. In *Supports for families with a disabled child: Collected papers from an International Cross-Cultural Conference.* New York: The Graduate School and University Center, The City University of New York.

Goodman, E. (1989). *Making sense*. New York: Atlantic Monthly Press.

HSRI/UCPA receive NIDRR grant on family support policy. (1986). *Family Support Bulletin, 1*(1), 2.

Johnson, S.H. (1979). *High risk parenting: Nursing assessment and strategies for the family at risk*. Philadelphia: J.P. Lippincott.

Kappel, B., Lusthaus, E., & Snow, J. (1989). Family support and services in Canada. In *Support for families with a disabled child: Collected papers from an International Cross-Cultural Conference*. New York: The Graduate School and University Center, The City University of New York.

Lipsky, D.K. (1985). A parental perspective on stress and coping. *American Journal of Orthopsychiatry, 55*(4), 614–617.

Lipsky, D.K. (1987). Introduction and overview. In D.K. Lipsky (Ed.), *Family supports for families with a disabled member* (pp. 5–11). New York: World Rehabilitation Fund.

Lipsky, D.K. (1989). The roles of parents. In D.K. Lipsky & A. Gartner (Eds.), *Beyond separate education: Quality education for all* (pp. 159–180). Baltimore: Paul H. Brookes Publishing Co.

McKaig, K. (1986). *Beyond the threshold: Families caring for their children who have significant developmental disabilities*. New York: Community Service Society of New York.

Miles, M. (1988). An information challenge. *International Rehabilitation Review, 39*(203), 6.

Mittler, P., & Russell, P. (1989). Support systems for families with a disabled child in the United Kingdom. In *Supports for families with a disabled child: Collected papers from an International Cross-Cultural Conference*. New York: The Graduate School and University Center, The City University of New York.

Odeck, A.A. (1989). Support systems for families with disabled children: Republic of Kenya. In *Supports for families with a disabled child: Collected papers from an International Cross-Cultural Conference*. New York: The Graduate School and University Center, The City University of New York.

Oi, F., Higuchi, K., & Takei, K. (1989). Support services for families with disabled children: Japan. In *Supports for families with a disabled child: Collected papers from an International Cross-Cultural Conference*. New York: The Graduate School and University Center, The City University of New York.

Riden, G., Wastberg, I.C., & Wendelholt, A. (1988). *Family support services in Sweden*. Unpublished manuscript.

Serpell, R. (1988). Igniting the process of mutual adaptation. *International Rehabilitation Review, 39*(2–3) 5–6.

Smith, F. (1987). UCPA Think Tank" identifies essential components of family support. *Family Support Bulletin, 1*(1), 4.

Speranza, R. (1989). Policies and support services for the family of the disabled person: Uruguay. In *Supports for families with a disabled child: Collected papers from an International Cross-Cultural Con-*

ference. New York: The Graduate School and University Center, The City University of New York.

Taylor, S.J., Knoll, J.A., Lehr, S., & Walker, P.M. (1989). Families for all children: Value-based services for children with disabilities and their families. In G.H.S. Singer & L.K. Irvin (Eds.), *Support for caregiving families: Enabling positive adaptation to disability* (pp. 41–53). Baltimore: Paul H. Brookes Publishing Co.

Turnbull, A.P., & Turnbull, H.R. (1989). *Work group on families. Leadership Institute on Community Integration.* Syracuse: Center on Human Policy.

Werner, D. (1988). Extension of the status quo or grassroots transformation? *International Rehabilitation Review, 39*(2–3), 5.

World Programme of Action Concerning Disabled Persons. (1983). New York: United Nations.

APPENDIX

Excerpts from *Disability, Society, and Social Change*—Principles and Objectives.

The Principles are:

1. People with disabilities are individuals who have the inherent right to respect for their human worth and dignity.
2. People with disabilities, whatever the origin, nature, type and degree of disability, have the same basic human rights as other members of Australian society.
3. People with disabilities have the same rights as other members of Australian society to realize their individual capacities for physical, social, emotional, and intellectual development.
4. People with disabilities have the same rights as other members of Australian society to services which will support their attaining a reasonable quality of life.
5. People with disabilities have the same right as other members of Australian society to participate in the decisions which affect their lives.
6. People with disabilities receiving services have the same right as other members of Australian society to receive those services in a manner which results in the least restriction of their rights and opportunities.
7. People with disabilities have the same right of pursuit of any grievance in relation to services as have other members of Australian society.

The Objectives are:

1. Services should have as their focus the achievement of positive outcomes for people with disabilities, such as increased independence, employment opportunities and integration into the community.
2. Services should contribute to ensuring that the conditions of the every-day life of people with disabilities are the same as, or as close as possible to norms and patterns which are valued in the general community.

From *Disability, society and social change.* (1988). Canberra, Australia: Commonwealth of Australia.

3. Services should be provided as part of local co-ordinated services systems and be integrated with services generally available to members of the community, whenever possible.

4. Services should be tailored to meet the individual needs and goals of the people with disabilities receiving those services.

5. Programs and services should be designed and administered so as to meet the needs of people with disabilities who experience a double disadvantage as a result of their sex, ethnic origin, or Aboriginality.

6. Programs and services should be designed and administered so as to promote recognition of the competence of, and enhance the image of, people with disabilities.

7. Programs and services should be designed and administered so as to promote the participation of people with disabilities in the life of the local community through maximum physical and social integration in that community.

8. Programs and services should be designed and administered so as to assure that no single organization providing services should exercise control over all or most aspects of the life of an individual with disabilities.

9. Organizations providing services, whether those services are provided specifically to people with disabilities or generally to members of the community, should be accountable to those people with disabilities who use their services, the advocates of such people, the Commonwealth and the community generally for the provision of information from which the quality of services can be judged.

10. Programs and services should be designed and administered so as to provide opportunities for people with disabilities to reach goals and enjoy lifestyles which are valued by the community generally and are appropriate to their chronological age.

11. Services should be designed and administered so as to ensure that people with disabilities have access to advocacy support where necessary to ensure adequate participation in decision-making about the services they receive.

12. Programs and services should be designed and administered so as to ensure that appropriate avenues exist for people with disabilities to raise and have resolved any grievances about services.

13. Services should be designed and administered so as to provide people with disabilities with, and encourage them to make use of, avenues for participating in the planning and operation of services which they receive and the Commonwealth and organizations should provide opportunities for consultation in relation to the development of major policy and program changes.

14. Programs and services should be designed and administered so as to respect the rights of people with disabilities to privacy and confidentiality.

Afterword

Following the Wingspread Conference, Doug Limbrick, a member of the Australian team and Director, Supported Accommodation Assistance Program, Department of Community Services and Health, Commonwealth of Australia, wrote us with a set of suggestions to implement the conference findings. While specific to the conference, they offer a widescale strategy for implementing a program of support for families with a child with a disability, and, as such, may have broader application. We present them, in that hope.

STRATEGY FOR IMPLEMENTATION OF CONFERENCE FINDINGS

OBJECTIVE

The objective of the strategy is to provide for children and youth with disabilities and their parents and families a set of supportive, goal directed services and programs to facilitate greater independence, freedom and a valued place in society.

PRINCIPLES AND VALUES

The strategy is based on a number of agreed principles and values. By and large these are principles which are widely accepted as those necessary to enhance the provision of services to families and persons with disabilities. The following principles underline the strategy:

All parents, families and young people with a disability should have access to appropriate services and supports.

Services to meet the needs of families and young people should be available regardless of residence, type of disability or other circumstances.

All services for families and young people with a disability should be provided as part of the community's general services wherever possible.

Services should be provided in a manner which maximises individual benefits and achievements, and enables families and young people to have a lifestyle which promotes personal development, growth and autonomy.

The options and choices available to families and disabled young people should be the same as those for the community generally.

Services should support and strengthen family structures and networks.

PRIORITIES

The following are the priorities put forward by the strategy to meet the needs of families and young people with a disability.

Reinforcing the Role of Families

Approaches need to be established which assist and reinforce the role of the family in the social development and participation of the young person with a disability in community life and uphold and support the family in normal activities, growth and development.

Importance of Community Living

Living within the community is a central goal for people with a disability. Participation in this community life is the expression of a person's community adjustment. The stimulation provided by community contacts provides, for the family members, including the person with a disability, social integration, personal identity and satisfaction in life experiences. Regardless of any support required on a periodic or continuing basis, the acceptance of this position is regarded as one of the priorities to be achieved.

Cultivation of Positive Community Perceptions of the Person with a Disability in Childhood and as an Adult

This process supports the point above. Positive community perceptions are among the most needed changes in support of a young person with a disability moving through childhood, adolescence and on to adult life. This process should begin in pre-school activities and particularly in school.

Reinforcing the Place of Community-Based Support Services

Learning to live within the community can best be achieved by young people with a disability when they experience life within the community, and the assistance they need is provided in the community. The perception of young people with a disability as a part of the wider society is also important in this experience. While specialised services will at times be required by some young people with a disability, community based services should be assisted to accept this role as part of the provision of assistance to all members of the community. Segregated specialised services should not be provided, without first pursuing the option of using and modifying, as necessary, community services for this role. Young people with a disability and their families should be assisted to use these services to the extent that they best meet their needs.

Ensuring that Generic Human Services Are Sensitive and Competent

The priorities above strongly advocate that community level services and experiences are an essential part of providing adequately for young people with a disability as they grow up. However, as with all services available to disadvantaged groups in our society, generic community services must be sensitive to the position and needs of young people with disabilities and their families. They must also be competent to provide appropriately for them.

PROCESSES

The processes proposed in the strategy for promoting the co-ordinated provision of services and supports to families and young people with a disability are set out below. The strategy emphasises the priorities and the processes needed to achieve the objectives and does not propose detailed programs. The development of the programs from the priorities and processes is left to individual countries.

Coordination

This has been an elusive aspect in most countries in the development and provision of services to people with disabilities and their families. Overcoming the existing difficulties in co-ordinating planning, development and delivery of services is an important part of this strategy. The importance of co-ordination across service areas (e.g., pre-school, home support, education, employment, community living), agencies in each service area, sectors in each service area (government and non-government), age levels and so on, is a key to efficiently and effectively implementing the strategy.

Co-ordination needs are such that there is not one solution to this problem. There needs to be an emphasis on co-ordination needs at each level of service. There are two specific ways that co-ordination can be improved, namely:

i. There is a need for governments and agencies to ensure appropriate co-ordination of legislation, programs and funding, in service delivery.
ii. There is a need to establish a mechanism to co-ordinate services for each family and individual with a disability. This could involve a family plan and/or an individual plan which maps out the options and solutions to providing assistance and services for each family or person from service to service and across service areas.

The lack of co-ordination frequently causes difficulties for families and individuals with a disability at the transition points in life. For example, when the young person moves from school to further study, training or employment. Co-ordination is therefore one of the central processes of the strategy.

The process of co-ordination raises the question of intergovernmental and interagency responsibilities. Across-government responsibilities implies clear agreement and definition by different levels of government of the responsibilities of each. The present array of services, benefits and supports available in many countries, however, does not indicate the presence of such agreements. Likewise, there is little evidence of across-agency agreement or division of responsibilities. Indeed many agencies provide parallel services, sometimes for similar groups, with little regard for the ensuing overlap. This frequently occurs in the context of providing an exclusive set of services to a specific group of people with disabilities on a total life basis.

Legislative Change

There is no underlying tradition in most countries of legislation covering the full range of assistance and services to all people with disabilities and their families. Legislation frequently covers only part of the population that could potentially benefit from whatever services are covered by the legislation. For example, legislation may only cover people with blindness, or adults but not children, or all types of disabilities except people with mental illness. There are many examples of this type of legislation.

Another legislative problem is simply an absence of legislation to support major difficulties encountered by families and their children with disabilities. The full range of issues to be considered includes the role of anti-discrimination, human rights and equal opportunity legislation in support of people with disabilities, the use of legislation to specify the objectives of funding and of services provided, and legislation which strengthens accountability arrangements, and helps to ensure the appropriateness and quality of provisions.

This component of the strategy requires an examination of existing legislation and proposes that legislation be employed to help ensure the services required by people with disabilities and their families are provided in such a way that the interests of the recipient are paramount, and that families and indi-

viduals are given maximum support in their quest for establishment within the community.

Personnel Preparation

Adequate training arrangements for personnel involved in
human services has for many years been considered an important component of service delivery. It is likewise considered
important to achieving the objective of the strategy. Although
there have been considerable developments in this area, especially in special education, there still remain significant
shortfalls in training in most countries.

While on the one hand there may be advanced or sophisti-
cated training programs in some program areas (e.g., education), on the other hand, there are often major deficiencies in
very basic training (e.g., community outreach workers, attendant carers, residential workers). A further difficulty is that
sometimes the training is adequate but the number of trained
personnel is deficient or inadequate numbers are hired.

In many instances simple training solutions are frequently
the most effective. For example, on the job or in-house training
for service delivery people with basic qualifications can be an
effective and efficient (little disruption) method of providing
additional skills to meet particular service needs. A phenomenon being encountered in some discipline areas in some countries is a movement towards overtraining. As personnel gain
additional qualifications, they frequently move away from
"hands-on" activities and seek higher paid positions. This can
provide a shortfall in service personnel and/or it can lead to a
steady creep in the minimum qualifications demanded for
front line service positions. Overqualified people tend to move
on more frequently, disrupting service delivery and relationships with the clients.

While there are a number of sides to the training issue, the
basic difficulty in most countries is a shortfall in the number of
trained personnel employed in these services.

Attitude Change

This is an important part of the strategy. Achievement of
positive attitudes towards people with disabilities and towards
their families is an integral part of full community integration.
While it is sometimes agreed that attitude change programs are

unsuccessful or take too long to have any impact, it is nonetheless true that community and individual attitudes and perceptions can prevent realisation or at least the full realisation of a goal.

Many countries experienced attempts at this process during 1981: International Year of Disabled Persons. While there have been varying reports about the success of these and subsequent campaigns, there appears to have been some impact in most places. We are now halfway through the UN Decade for Disabled Persons; an important goal for the remaining half would be achievement of a significant shift in community attitudes.

Some people argue that the most effective method of achieving positive community attitudes is to provide the programs and supports that enable people with disabilities to be integrated participating members of the community. This enables the community to see these people living normal lives, thus changing perceptions.

A further method advocated is for service groups, interest groups and governments (at all levels) to endorse and actively promote clear philosophical statements which advocate a valued place in society for people with a disability.

Clearly all these processes are important in this endeavour.

Provision of Data and Support for Research

The need for good data in most areas of human services, including services for people with disabilities, has long been recognised as important. Co-ordination, planning and the provision of services must be based on adequate data. The full effectiveness of services, including the mounting of an adequate case for additional resources, can be impeded without data. Further efforts to obtain this information for all stages of the process are justified and are an important part of the overall strategy.

The same comments apply to an adequate level of research to support and foster new methods, programs, models and solutions. A key requirement here is to ensure that the findings of these efforts are translated into everyday practice so that the impact can be as far reaching as possible. All too frequently this is overlooked and good research findings take years to find their way into service provision.

HOW TO IMPLEMENT THIS STRATEGY

This section looks at the major methods of implementing the strategy. As stated previously, it is not presented as a list of suggested new programs or program needs, although, of course, individual countries may find it necessary to implement new programs to achieve the objectives set out in the strategy.

Setting Priorities

An important first step to implementation is the setting of priorities within existing services and between existing services and proposed services.

The priorities, as implied in the previous two sections, are:

A priority to community-based services and programs

A priority to attitude change and development and to the development of sensitivity in service provision

A priority to co-ordination of available services and programs, providing for people with a disability and their families a clear definition of agency responsibilities

A priority to reinforce the role of families of people with a disability

A priority to support activities, rights, roles, responsibilities and services with comprehensive legislation

A priority for improved preparation of service personnel

A priority for establishment of a data base to inform and support further development and to aid allocation of scarce resources

A priority to support research and demonstration activity and a commitment to ensure that outcomes are translated into everyday practice

Better Use of Existing Resources

Human services in most countries suffer from a scarcity of resources for expansion and further development. The strategy proposed here recognises this and recommends that re-direction of existing resources is one method to support implementation. One way of achieving this is to look at existing services to see if they are still appropriate and relevant or if they might be delivered in a more efficient manner. With changes in society, changes in the needs of people with disabilities and their families, changes to the range of generic services, etc. many existing services may no longer be appropriate. Any re-direction of resources is, of course, a difficult process and will need to be undertaken in a planned and sensitive way to ensure continuity of support.

Provision of Co-operative Services

The move from segregated to community-level services also supports the concept of co-operative programs and services provided by and for people with disabilities and their families. Various specialist and generic agencies can co-operate to deliver supports, services and programs to achieve the objectives of this strategy. To implement and advance this approach will require specific support for these co-operative ventures. There is a need for this development to be encouraged and supported by policy change and revised funding arrangements.

Information Provision

This strategy statement emphasizes the need for information to the community, to service providers, and especially to people with a disability and their families. The availability of information which is meaningful and sensitive, and supportive of the desire by people with a disability to live and work in the community as other citizens, is central to the success of the strategy. This is therefore an important means of implementing the strategy. Information dissemination cannot be the responsibility of any one agency, although specialised agencies established for this task should take a predominant role. It is, however, a task for all agencies and for people with disabilities and their organisations to ensure that public information, which develops positive community perceptions of and attitudes toward people with a disability, and information providing knowledge and understanding of the services and provisions in support of people with a disability, is available and utilised.

Index

Page numbers followed by "*t*" indicate tables.

ABCX Model, 68–69
Adaptation
coping strategies for, 69
of families, 62, 65–70
models of, 68–69
Advocacy, parental, 73
"Aesthetic anxiety," 44, 87
African-Americans, 46–47
Aid to Families with Dependent
Children, 120
American Coalition of Citizens
with Disabilities, 41
Americans with Disabilities Act,
121
Amniocentesis, 19
Anger, parental, 62
Asylums, 39
Attitudinal influences, 41–43
Australia
Child Disability Allowance in,
102
disability information systems
in, 128
Disability Service Act of,
100–101
education in, 101–102,
137–138
emotional support in,
166–167
employment services in, 175
financial assistance in,
99–102
Home and Community Care
Act of, 101
housing in, 176
issues identified for attention
in, 188–189
legislation in, 100
recreation services in, 176

respite services in, 157
responsible federal departments in, 100
state and territory programs
in, 100

Begging, 22–23
Blindness
accommodative adjustment to,
24
cultural attitudes toward, 19,
24
legal, 6
"river blindness," 24
socialization processes and, 4
Bodily perfection, 2
Brain-injured child, 65–67

Canada
Charter of Rights and Freedoms in, 104–105
disability information systems
in, 128–129
early intervention in, 138–139
education in, 103, 138–142
emotional support in,
167–168
employment services in,
176–177
family support in, 105
federal responsibilities in,
102–103
financial assistance in,
102–105
housing in, 177
institutional vs. community-
based services in, 104

Canada—*continued*
  interprovincial program varia-
    tions in, 103
  issues identified for attention
    in, 189–190
  legislation in, 103
  program funding in, 103
  provincial responsibilities in,
    103–104
  respite services in, 157–158
  service delivery in, 104
Chinese-Americans, 46–47
Civil Rights Movement, 40
Community-based services,
  185–187
  moral responsibility for,
    186
  vs. traditional model, 186
Co-ordination of services,
  216–217
Coping-Health Inventory for Parents, 65
Coping strategies, 69
Cultural views, 17–50
  on aesthetics of disabilities,
    43–46
  of Africans, 34, 34t
  cross-cultural comparisons of,
    46–48
  infanticide and, 22
  literary, 36–38
  of mental retardation, 4
  North Korean, 17–18
  shame- vs. guilt-oriented, 22
  social resources and, 38–41
  of societal place of disabled
    persons, 41–43
  toward blindness, 19, 24
  toward deafness, 18–19,
    25–28
  toward disability, 2–5
  toward Down syndrome, 18,
    19
  toward women with dis-
    abilities, 28–30
  transfer between countries of,
    186–187
  work vs. need systems and, 5

Deaf persons
  community inclusion of, 18
  culture of, 86
  developmental capacity of,
    25–26
  historical roles of, 25–28
  Justinian Code about, 25
  language of, 25
  on Martha's Vineyard, 18–19,
    27, 30
  sense of identity of, 86
  stereotypes of, 33–34
  traits attributed to, 34–35,
    35t
  use of sign language by,
    27–28
Denial, 61–62
Developmental Disabilities Act of
  1970, 122
Developmental hierarchies,
  30–36
Disabilities
  cultural attitudes toward, 2–5
  cultural definitions of, 21, 41
  different disciplines' views of,
    3–4
    economic, 3
    political, 3
    psychological, 3
    sociological, 3–4
  distributive dilemma and, 5–6
  environmental mitigation of, 41
  genuine vs. artificial, 23
  information systems about,
    127–135
  medical model of, 42
  special treatment for persons
    with, 4
  state-of-the-art vs. traditional
    perceptions of, 64, 65t
  vs. handicaps, 2
Disability, Society, and Social
  Change, 211–213
  objectives of, 211–212
  principles of, 211
Disabled persons
  advocacy groups for, 41
  aversion to, 44, 87

conceptualizations of societal place of, 41–43
cultural attitudes toward, 21–50, *see also* Cultural views
cultural roles of, 22–23
difficulty in defining, 1
education of, 137–153, *see also* Education
expectations for, 13
families of, 57–89, *see also* Families; Parents
human nature of, 21, 43–46
integration vs. segregation of, 9–11
"least restrictive alternatives" for, 12–13
legislation for, 40
literary images of, 36–38
myths vs. realities about, 8–15
"primitiveness" of, 32–34
rights and obligations of, 207–208
sense of identity of, 84–88
society's "bargain" with, 43–44
subculture of, 86–87
support services for, 8–9
who live in outlying areas, 11–12
women, 28–30
Distributive systems, 5–6
Divorce, 70
Doctor shopping, 59, 61
Down, J.L.H., 32–33
Down syndrome, 18, 19

Education, 137–153
in Australia, 101–102, 137–138
in Canada, 103, 138–142
in Israel, 142–144
in Japan, 144–145
in Kenya, 145
in Sweden, 145
in United Kingdom, 146–150

in United States, 151–152
in Uruguay, 152–153
Education for All Handicapped Children Act (PL 94-142), 40, 73, 151
Education of the Handicapped Act Amendments (PL 99-457), 134, 151
Emotional support, 165–174
in Australia, 166–167
in Canada, 167–168
factors affecting extent of need for, 166
in Israel, 168–169
in Japan, 169–170
in Kenya, 170
in Sweden, 170
in United Kingdom, 171–172
in United States, 172–174
universal need for, 165–166
in Uruguay, 174
Employment services, 175–184
in Australia, 175
in Canada, 176–177
in Israel, 177
in Japan, 109–110, 178–179
in Kenya, 179
in Sweden, 180
in United Kingdom, 181
in United States, 181–182
in Uruguay, 183–184
Environment
effect on impairments, 41
interaction of disabled person with, 43

Families
adaptations of, 62, 65–70
alikeness of, 57–58, 166
coping strategies of, 69
decision-making rights of, 14–15
different perspectives within, 58
emotional support for, 165–174, *see also* Emotional support

Families—*continued*
  financial assistance for, 98,
    see also Financial
    assistance
  labeling parents in, 58–63
  life cycle needs in, 70–73, 72*t*
  needs of, 15
  providing information for,
    127–135
  respite services for, 155–163,
    see also Respite services
  single-parent, 70
  stress theory for, 68
  stresses on, 199
  theoretical approaches to
    study of, 67
  traditional vs. state-of-the-art
    roles of, 66*t*
  transactional model of, 68
  see also Parents
Family Adaptability and Cohesion Scales, 65
Family Adjustment and Adaptation Response Model, 68
Family Inventory of Life Events
  and Changes, 66
Family support
  characteristics of effective pro-
    grams for, 206–207
  conceptual underpinnings of,
    200–201
  definition of, 199–200
  essential components of, 205
  factors affecting program de-
    velopment for, 200
  need for flexibility in, 200
  principles of planning for, 206
  strategy for implementation
    of, 213–221, *see also* Im-
    plementation strategies
  traditional vs. state-of-the-art
    practices for, 201,
    202*t*–205*t*
Financial assistance, 97–125
  in Australia, 99–102
  in Canada, 102–105
  common trends in, 125
  eligibility for, 97–98

  employment-based, 97, 99
  governmental level of, 98–99
  in Israel, 105–108
  in Japan, 108–111
  in Kenya, 111–113
  in Sweden, 113–115
  types of, 97–98
  in United Kingdom, 115–120
  in United States, 120–123
  in Uruguay, 124
  variations in, 97, 125
Freud, S., 32
Friends, 89

Generational continuity, 87

Housing
  in Australia, 176
  in Canada, 177
  in Israel, 177
  in Japan, 179
  in Kenya, 180
  in Sweden, 180
  in United Kingdom, 116, 181
  in United States, 182–183
  in Uruguay, 184
Human nature, 21, 43–46

Identity, 84–88
Implementation strategies,
  215–223
  methods of, 220–221
  objective of, 215
  principles and values of, 216
  priorities of, 216–218
  processes of, 218–221
    attitude change, 220–221
    co-ordination, 218–219
    legislation, 219–220
    personnel preparation, 220
    research, 221
Individualized Education Program, 133–134, 151
Infanticide, 22

Information, 221
  formal systems for, 127–135,
    see also specific countries
  parental need for, 76
Institutionalization
  alternatives to, 64
  development of, 39
  parents' refusal of, 63–64
Intelligence
  definition of, 31–32
  developmental hierarchies of,
    30–36
Iranians, 48–49
Israel
  Arabs in Israel, 46, 47, 158,
    169, 190
  attitudes toward Iranian pa-
    tients in, 48–49
  disability information systems
    in, 129–130
  education in, 142–144
  eligibility for assistance in,
    107
  emotional support in,
    168–169
  employment services in, 177
  family impact of disabled child
    in, 62
  family support in, 107–108
  financial assistance in,
    105–108
  housing in, 178
  issues identified for attention
    in, 190–191
  legislation in, 106
  Ministry of Labor and Social
    Affairs of, 105–106
  National Insurance Institute
    of, 106
  National Workers Sick Fund
    of, 106
  non-government support in,
    107
  parent training in, 143
  recreation services in, 178
  Rehabilitation Administration
    of, 106–107
  respite services in, 158

  views about disability in,
    47–48

Japan
  disability information systems
    in, 130–131
  early intervention services in,
    109
  education in, 144–145
  emotional support in,
    169–170
  employment services in,
    109–110, 178–179
  family support in, 110
  financial assistance in,
    108–111
  health insurance system of,
    108–109
  housing in, 179
  issues identified for attention
    in, 191–193
  legislation in, 108–110
  Maternal and Child Health
    Law in, 109
  Ministry of Health and Welfare
    in, 109–110
  recreation services in, 179
  respite services in, 158
  service delivery in, 110
  subsidized transportation
    costs in, 110–111
Jung, C., 32
Justinian Code, 25

Kenya
  children's services in, 112
  Civitan Foundation, 132, 145,
    180, 193
  DANIDA/Kenya program in,
    112–113
  disability information systems
    in, 131–132
  education in, 145
  emotional support in, 170
  employment services in, 179

Kenya—*continued*
  financial assistance in,
    111–113
  housing in, 180
  Institute of Special Education
    in, 113
  issues identified for attention
    in, 193–194
  Ministry of Culture and Social
    Services of, 111–113
  non-governmental agencies in,
    112
  recreation services in, 180
  respite services in, 158
  vocational rehabilitation in,
    111

Language, 25
Leadership Institute on Commu-
    nity Integration, 64
"Least restrictive alternatives,"
    12–13
Legislation, 219–220
  in Australia, 100–102
  in Canada, 103
  in Israel, 106
  in Japan, 108–110
  in Kenya, 145
  parents' roles in development
    of, 64
  in Sweden, 113, 115
  in United Kingdom, 117–119
  in Uruguay, 124
  in United States, 40, 120
Life cycle needs, 70–73, 72*t*

Martha's Vineyard, deaf persons
    on, 18–19, 27, 30
Medicaid, 120, 122
Medicare, 120
Mexican-Americans, 47
Myths, 8–15

Parent-professional part-
    nerships, 78–84

essentials of, 80
guidelines for development of,
    83–84
harmful effects of, 78–79
requirements for success of,
    79–80
roles in, 80–82
traditional vs. state-of-the-art
    views of, 80, 81*t*–82*t*
Parent Training and Information
    Programs, 134
Parents
  advocacy by, 73
  anger of, 62
  denial by, 61–62
  emotional support for,
    165–174, *see also* Emo-
    tional support
  entrepreneur concept of, 78
  informational needs of, 76
  instrumental vs. expressive
    roles of, 67–68
  involvement of, 73–78
    in communicating, 74*t*–75*t*
    critiques of, 76–77
    in learning at home,
      74*t*–75*t*
    in parenting, 74*t*–75*t*
    in representing other par-
      ents, 74*t*–75*t*
    in volunteering, 74*t*–75*t*
  labeling of, 58–63, 165–166
  "new philosophy of parentol-
    ogy," 77
  perspectives of, 58
  rejection of child by, 62
  responses to attitudes and ser-
    vices in United States,
    63–64
  self-narratives of, 60
  sense of identity imparted by,
    84–88
  single-parent families, 70
  social pathology paradigm of
    behavior of, 59–60
  sorrow and joy of, 61
  traditional vs. state-of-the-art
    roles of, 66*t*

training programs for, 80–82
visiting multiple doctors by,
      59, 61
see also Families
Permanency planning, 66*t*
Persons with mental retardation
   cultural definitions of, 4
   effect of cultural complexity
      on, 30
   as parents, 88
   parents' refusal for institu-
      tionalization of, 63–64
   self-perception of, 19–20
   sexuality of, 31
   societal exclusion of, 2
Poor Laws, 38–39
Portage Model for Home Teach-
      ing, 148
"Primitive mind," 31

Recreation services
   in Australia, 176
   in Israel, 178
   in Japan, 179
   in Kenya, 180
   in Sweden, 180
   in United Kingdom, 181
   in United States, 183
   in Uruguay, 184
Rehabilitation Act of 1973 (PL
      93-112), 40, 121
Rejection, of child by parents,
      62
Research, 219
Respite services, 155–163
   in Australia, 157
   balance between family and
      child benefits of, 155–156
   in Canada, 157–158
   cultural appropriateness of,
      162
   current developments in, 162
   definition of, 156
   institutional settings for, 162
   in Israel, 158
   in Japan, 158
   in Kenya, 158

limitations of, 162
   in Sweden, 159
   in United Kingdom, 159–160
   in United States, 160–161
   in Uruguay, 161
   variations in, 156
Retirement age, 6

Segregation
   development of institutions
      for, 39–40
   vs. community participation,
      9–11
Separation/divorce, 70
Service planning, 206
Sexuality, 31, 87
Siblings' roles, 66*t*
Sickle cell anemia, 18
Sign language, 27–28
Single-parent families, 70
Social welfare provisions,
      97–125
   in Australia, 99–102
   in Canada, 102–105
   common trends in, 125
   in Israel, 105–108
   in Japan, 108–111
   in Kenya, 111–113
   in Sweden, 113–115
   in United Kingdom, 115–120
   in United States, 120–123
   in Uruguay, 124
   variations in, 97, 125
Supplemental Security Income,
      121–122
Sweden, 187
   Act on Special Services for In-
      tellectually Handicapped
      Persons of, 115
   disability information systems
      in, 132
   education in, 145
   emotional support in, 170
   employment services in, 180
   financial assistance in,
      113–115
   housing in, 180

Sweden—*continued*
immigrants to, 194–195
integrated services in, 114
issues identified for attention
    in, 194–195
national health insurance in,
    114–115
parental insurance in, 114
public child care in, 114
recreation services in, 180
respite services in, 159
responsibility for services in,
    113–114

United Kingdom
disability allowances in,
    118–119
disability information systems
    in, 133
early intervention in, 147–148
education in, 146–150
emotional support in,
    171–172
employment services in, 116,
    181
family support in, 118
financial assistance in,
    115–120
fragmentation of services in,
    116–117
housing in, 116, 181
issues identified for attention
    in, 195–197
legislation in, 117–119
national curriculum in,
    149–150
National Health Service of,
    116
Portage Model for Home Teach-
    ing in, 148
recreation services in, 181
report on families with dis-
    abled children in,
    119–120
respite services in, 159–160
responsibility for services in,
    115–116
Social Security Act of, 119

Warnock Committee in,
    146–147
United States
Aid to Families with Depen-
    dent Children program in,
    120
Developmental Disabilities Act
    of, 122
disability information systems
    in, 133–134
education in, 151–152
emotional support in,
    172–174
employment services in,
    181–182
ethnic minorities' views to-
    ward disability in, 46–47
financial assistance in,
    120–123
food assistance programs in,
    121
housing in, 182–183
issues identified for attention
    in, 197–198
legislation in, 120
Medicaid in, 120, 122
Medicare in, 120
parents' responses to attitudes
    and services in, 63–64
private programs in, 123
recreation services in, 183
respite services in, 160–161
retirement age in, 6
state programs in, 123
Supplemental Security Income
    in, 121–122
transition planning in, 182
Vocational Rehabilitation Act
    of, 123
Uruguay
centrality of family in, 124
disability information systems
    in, 134–135
education in, 152–153
emotional support in, 174
employment services in,'
    183–184
family support in, 124
financial assistance in, 124

housing in, 184
issues identified for attention
    in, 198–199
legislation in, 124
recreation services in, 184
respite services in, 161
Social Security system of, 124

Vocational Rehabilitation Act,
    123

Women with disabilities, 28–30